HEALTH AND DEPRIVATION:
Inequality and the North

HEALTH AND DEPRIVATION

Inequality and the North

Peter Townsend, Peter Phillimore
and Alastair Beattie

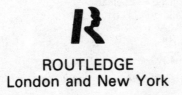

ROUTLEDGE
London and New York

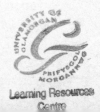

1111443 6

First published in 1988 by
Croom Helm Ltd, Provident House,
Burrell Row, Beckenham, Kent BR3 1AT

Reprinted 1989 by Routledge
11 New Fetter Lane, London EC4P 4EE
29 West 35th Street, New York, NY 10001

Printed and bound in Great Britain by
Biddles Ltd, Guildford and King's Lynn

British Library Cataloguing in Publication Data
Townsend, Peter, 1928—
    Health and deprivation: inequality
    and the north.
    1. Social medicine — England
    I. Title II. Phillimore, Peter
    III. Beattie, Alastair
    613   RA418.3.G7
    ISBN 0-415-04298-4

Library of Congress Cataloging in Publication Data also available

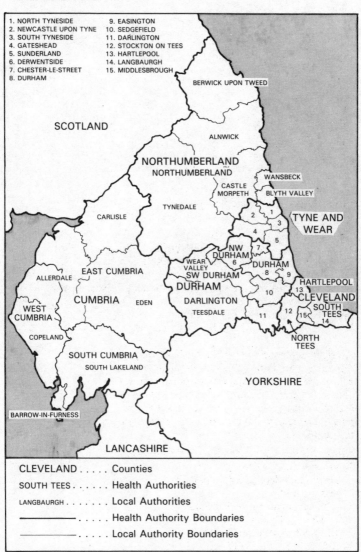

HEALTH AND LOCAL AUTHORITIES
IN THE NORTHERN REGION

1. NORTH TYNESIDE
2. NEWCASTLE UPON TYNE
3. SOUTH TYNESIDE
4. GATESHEAD
5. SUNDERLAND
6. DERWENTSIDE
7. CHESTER-LE-STREET
8. DURHAM
9. EASINGTON
10. SEDGEFIELD
11. DARLINGTON
12. STOCKTON ON TEES
13. HARTLEPOOL
14. LANGBAURGH
15. MIDDLESBROUGH

SCOTLAND

BERWICK UPON TWEED

ALNWICK

NORTHUMBERLAND
NORTHUMBERLAND

WANSBECK

CASTLE
MORPETH

BLYTH VALLEY

TYNEDALE

CARLISLE

TYNE AND
WEAR

NW
DURHAM

WEAR
VALLEY

SW DURHAM

DURHAM

DURHAM

EAST CUMBRIA

ALLERDALE

HARTLEPOOL

CUMBRIA

EDEN

DARLINGTON

CLEVELAND

WEST
CUMBRIA

TEESDALE

SOUTH
TEES

COPELAND

NORTH
TEES

SOUTH CUMBRIA
SOUTH LAKELAND

YORKSHIRE

BARROW-IN-FURNESS

LANCASHIRE

CLEVELAND . . . . . Counties

SOUTH TEES . . . . . . Health Authorities

LANGBAURGH . . . . Local Authorities

———— . . . . . Health Authority Boundaries

———— . . . . . Local Authority Boundaries

Contents

List of Figures   vii
List of Tables   ix
Preface   xiii

Part One: The Approach

1.   Introduction: Aims, Concepts and Theories   3
1.1   Concepts and Models of Health   6
1.2   The Contemporary Case for a Fresh Approach   11

2.   The Northern Region and the North–South Divide   18
2.1   Population and Economy   19
2.2   North and South: Changes in 50 years   25
2.3   North and South: The Gap Today   27

3.   Indicators of Health and Deprivation   30
3.1   The Construction of a Measure of Health   30
3.2   The Construction of a Measure of Deprivation   34
3.3   The Ward as a Unit of Analysis   38

Part Two: Description

4.   The Distribution of Poor Health in the Northern
      Region   43
4.1   Overall Poor Health   45
4.2   Mortality   47
4.3   Permanent Sickness and Disability   60
4.4   Low Birthweight   62

5.   The Prevalence of Deprivation in the Northern
      Region   66
5.1   Overall Deprivation   66
5.2   Individual Measures of Deprivation   70

6.   The Link Between Health and Deprivation   74
6.1   The Range of Variation within the Region: Overall
      Health   74
6.2   Premature Mortality   84
6.3   Life in the Poorest Wards   88

Part Three: Explanation

7. Occupational Class and the Explanation of Health
    Inequalities   95
7.1 The Treatment of Class   95
7.2 Class Gradients in Mortality and Low Birthweight   96
7.3 Excess Mortality and Occupational Class   101

8. Material Deprivation and the Explanation of Health
    Inequalities   107
8.1 The Strength of the Association between Health and
    Deprivation   107
8.2 Predictable and Paradoxical Patterns of Health   112
8.3 Explaining Inequalities in Health: Regression Analysis   116
8.4 Explaining Mortality in Cleveland and Tyne and
    Wear: Regression Analysis   121

9. The Widening Mortality Gap in Britain and the North   128
9.1 The Presentation of the Evidence   139
9.2 The North in Relation to National Trends   145
9.3 Conclusion   149

10. Conclusions   151
10.1 Aims and Concepts   152
10.2 Findings   153

Notes   159
Glossary   161

Appendices

1   Data Sources, Definitions of the Variables and
    Handling the Data   163
2   The Creation of Summary Variables: The Z-Score
    Technique   165
3   Estimating the Number of Deaths due to an Area's
    Occupational Class Structure   166
4   Urban Areas: Definition   167
5   Additional Tables and Figures   168
6   Ranking of Wards on the Overall Health Index
References   199
Index   206

Figures

2.1 The distribution by age of all deaths under 75 years   26
4.1 Overall health. Proportion of each district's population living in wards ranked among the best and worst fifth in the Northern Region   46
4.2 Premature mortality. Proportion of each district's population living in wards ranked among the best and worst fifth in the Northern Region   48
4.3a Bloc of 15 wards in Cleveland (south bank of River Tees) with very high premature mortality   51
4.3b Bloc of six wards in Newcastle and Gateshead with very high premature mortality   51
4.4 Bloc of 22 wards in East Durham (chiefly Easington district) with high female premature mortality   53
4.5 Bloc of seven wards in West Cumbria with high premature mortality   54
4.6 The distribution by age of all deaths under 75 years in selected areas and for selected periods   59
4.7 Permanent sickness. Proportion of each district's population living in wards ranked among the best and worst fifth in the Northern Region   61
4.8 Low birthweight. Proportion of each district's population living in wards ranked among the best and worst fifth in the Northern Region   63
5.1 Overall deprivation. Proportion of each district's population living in wards ranked among the best and worst fifth in the Northern Region   69
6.1 The structure of inequality in the Northern Region: wards ranked on Overall Health Index   76
7.1 Standardising mortality for occupational class across the Northern Region: actual and predicted patterns compared, 1981–3   104
8.1 The relationship between health and deprivation in the Northern Region   109
A5.1 Unemployment. Proportion of each district's population living in wards ranked among the best and worst fifth in the Northern Region   168

A5.2 Car ownership. Proportion of each district's
population living in wards ranked among the best and
worst fifth in the Northern Region   169
A5.3 Overcrowding. Proportion of each district's
population living in wards ranked among the best and
worst fifth in the Northern Region   170
A5.4 Home ownership. Proportion of each district's
population living in wards ranked among the best and
worst fifth in the Northern Region   171

Tables

2.1 Age standardised mortality from all causes in 1980   21
2.2 The regional distribution of sickness and invalidity in Britain   22
2.3 Regional and district mortality: the Northern Region compared with the South-East and South-West Regions   24
2.4 SMRs (Standardised Mortality Ratios) for all causes 1979–80, 1982–3 for manual and non-manual occupations by region, men aged 20–64. Ranking of regions by manual SMR/non-manual SMR   25
2.5 North and South: some indicators of living standards   28
4.1 The twelve wards with the worst and best overall health in the Northern Region with populations over 3,000   44
4.2 Premature mortality in Tyne and Wear and Cleveland: based on ward groupings by district, 1981–3 deaths   49
4.3 Premature mortality (0–64) in five areas of the Northern Region, 1981–3: SMRs by selected causes   56
4.4 Trends in mortality in England and Wales   57
4.5 Low birthweight in Tyne and Wear and Cleveland, based on ward groupings by district, 1982–4 births   65
5.1 The twelve wards with the most and least Overall Deprivation in the Northern Region with populations over 3,000   67
6.1 Health and deprivation for ward groupings based on ranking of wards by Overall Health Index   77
6.2 Health and deprivation for urban and non-urban ward groupings based on ranking of wards by Overall Health Index   79
6.3 Health and deprivation in the local authorities of the Northern Region   80
6.4 Health and deprivation in the parliamentary constituencies of the Northern Region   82
6.5 Health and deprivation for ward groupings based on ranking of wards by persons 0–64 SMR   85

6.6 Mortality by cause of death. SMRs for deaths between 0 and 64 for ward groupings based on ranking of wards by persons 0–64 SMRs 87

7.1 Crude death rates (per 1,000 population) by occupational class for economically active men aged 16–64 in the Northern Region. Ward groupings (worst and best) based on ranking of wards by persons 0–64 SMR 97

7.2 Crude death rates by occupational class (non-manual and manual) and cause of death for economically active men aged 16–64 in the Northern Region. Worst and best quintile of wards ranked on persons 0–64 SMR 100

7.3 Low birthweight by occupational class in the Northern Region. Ward groupings based on ranking of wards by low birthweight (proportion of live births under 2,800 gm). 10% sample 102

7.4 Standardising mortality for occupational class in the 25% of wards with highest mortality in each district in Cleveland and Tyne and Wear, 1981–3: actual and predicted patterns compared 105

8.1 The relationship between the health and deprivation indicators for the Northern Region: Spearman rank correlation coefficients (678 wards) 108

8.2 The relationship between Overall Deprivation and each of the health indicators in the 29 local authorities of the Northern Region: Spearman rank correlation coefficients 110

8.3 Regressions of Overall Health Index separately on deprivation and class indicators for each Northern Region county: proportion of variance in overall health explained by each regression 118

8.4 The relationship between premature mortality and the deprivation indicators in Cleveland and Tyne and Wear combined: correlation coefficients 122

8.5 Assessing mortality in the light of deprivation in Cleveland and Tyne and Wear 123

8.6 Comparison of mortality taking account of occupational class and deprivation in three ward clusters 125

9.1 Mortality of men by occupational class over five decades (SMRs — England and Wales) 129

9.2   Mortality of married and single women by
      occupational class over two decades (SMRs —
      England and Wales)   130
9.3   Mortality rates per 100,000 and as a percentage of
      rates for occupational Classes I and II combined
      (1949–83, England and Wales, men and married
      women)   131
9.4   Trends in male mortality by class 1970–83 (England
      and Wales)   133
9.5a SMRs by cause, rich and poor classes: Great Britain
      (all men)   134
9.5b SMRs by cause, rich and poor classes: Great Britain
      (all women)   136
9.6   Mortality of men and women by occupational class,
      Britain and the Northern Region (SMRs 1979–80,
      1982–3)   145
9.7   Numbers of observed and expected deaths by
      occupational class, Northern Region, 1979–80 and
      1982–3   146
9.8   Mortality of men and women in different regions of
      Britain, 1979–80 and 1982–3   146
9.9   Mortality of men aged 20–64 and married women
      aged 20–59, direct age standardised mean annual
      death rates (per 1,000 population), 1979–80 and
      1982–3   147
9.10 SMRs for all causes, 1979–80 and 1982–3 by region   148
9.11 Trends in male mortality in the North, 1970–2,
      1979–80 and 1982–3   148
A5.1 Health and deprivation for ward groupings based on
      ranking of wards by permanent sickness   172
A5.2 Health and deprivation for ward groupings based on
      ranking of wards by low birthweight   173
A5.3 Health and deprivation for ward groupings based on
      ranking of wards by persons 0–64 SMR   174
A5.4 Selected avoidable deaths. SMRs for deaths between
      0–64 years for ward groupings based on ranking of
      wards by persons 0–64 SMR for all causes   175
A5.5 Avoidable deaths in Tyne and Wear and Cleveland:
      SMRs for the worst quarter of wards in each district
      for deaths between 0–64 years, 1981–3 inclusive   176
A5.6 Relationships within the two sets of variables:
      Spearman rank correlation coefficients (678 wards)   176

A5.7 The relationship between Overall Health and the deprivation and class indicators in each Northern Region county: Spearman rank correlation coefficients 177

A5.8 Regressions of Overall Health Index on deprivation and class indicators for each Northern Region county: proportion of variance in overall health explained by each regression 178

Preface

This book presents new evidence of inequalities in health found among populations or communities in different areas of the North of England, relates that evidence to long-term trends taking place in patterns of health in Britain as a whole, and explores how far health inequalities can be explained by variations in material deprivation. More than three million people live in the Northern Region, and their homes are distributed among 678 electoral wards. The differences between the populations of each of these wards lie at the heart of this study. Our object is to map the health differences and go on to find how far they are matched by differences in material and social conditions. The argument that health and wealth, or ill-health and deprivation, are highly correlated is an old one, but it is one which deserves fresh scrutiny in today's changed conditions. The research was undertaken between 1984 and 1986. This book is an updated, heavily revised and extended version of a report entitled 'Inequalities in Health in the Northern Region' which was produced jointly for more limited distribution by the Northern Regional Health Authority and the Department of Social Administration of the University of Bristol in 1986.

In 1980 the research working group on 'Inequalities in Health' under Sir Douglas Black found, after a careful review of many studies, that while genetic and cultural or behavioural explanations played their part, the predominant or governing explanation for inequalities in health lay in the material circumstances and conditions of people's lives, summarised by the concept of material deprivation. The group spelled out the consequences for policy, which ranged far beyond the scope of the work of the Department of Health and Social Security (DHSS), and also for statistical and scientific research. In the last seven years this thesis has gathered momentum. The number of area studies of health has multiplied and studies of unemployment, work conditions, environmental pollution, low income and specific occupations now amount to a formidable array of evidence. This evidence is also taken very seriously in a number of other industrial countries and has led to important initiatives on the part of the World Health Organisation. Thirty-three member countries of the European office of that organisation, including Britain, have agreed health targets for the year 2000, the first of which is equity in health, defined operationally as the achievement of a reduction of at least 25 per cent in the differences in health status between groups within countries and between countries by that year.

In focussing on the association between material deprivation and ill-health, we do not claim to be offering an exhaustive explanation for present health inequalities: the nature of the available evidence does not allow that to be attempted. One small, technical reason is that our subsequent analysis covers only those aspects of deprivation which can be extracted from official statistics. Inevitably, therefore, our assessment of the importance of material conditions of life (as well as of the criteria of health at our disposal) is incomplete. A more important reason is that health is affected by so many different influences, interacting in complex and still only partially understood ways, that we would not wish for a moment to deny that factors other than those we have highlighted in this study also help to shape the health of the population. However, although patterns of health in the community cannot be reduced to patterns of deprivation, as if the two were synonymous, it remains certain that variations in health cannot be understood without overriding emphasis being given to material conditions of life.

In the current debate about the causes of health differences between areas or social groups, a sharp distinction is often made between social or environmental factors influencing health, and those over which the individual has some control or choice. Diet, exercise and smoking are the obvious instances. The impact of life-style on health falls outside the scope of this study, but two observations need to be made. The first is that proponents of the individualistic approach consistently overlook the fact that smoking and eating habits, as well as the amount of exercise taken by people, are far from being activities determined solely by individual choice. Diet is profoundly influenced by cultural or local social customs, informal and formal education, the availability as well as price of goods in local markets, advertising, recipes and fashions recommended by the media, and decisions taken by farmers and the manufacturers of food products as well as by Government. Similar considerations apply to other behaviour, like physical exercise, smoking, and drinking. In other words, what is attributed to individual choice is in fact substantially shaped by powerful economic and social forces, the goods and facilities that are immediately available and level of income (among recent discussions of this theme, see Hart, 1986).

The second observation is that, contrary to some stereotypes of the way low-income families handle their money, there is evidence that they obtain necessary nutrients more efficiently at less cost than do richer families (Cole-Hamilton and Lang, 1986). Even so, such families do not have incomes large enough to buy the kind of diet recommended for health: so the adequacy or otherwise of household diet — which is supposed to epitomise the way in which the individual can crucially determine his or her own health prospects — depends substantially on the income available to the family and other facets of material deprivation.

While the primary subject-matter of this book is the link between poor health and material deprivation within the 678 wards of England's Northern Region, a closely related secondary theme is the link between poor health and occupational class. This link is examined regionally but also nationally. As we will show in subsequent pages (especially in Chapters 8 and 9), the analysis of deprivation helps to explain idiosyncracies in the variation by area of poor health which cannot be explained by a crude categorisation of populations by occupational class. This has major implications for scientific enquiry. However, the belated publication of the latest Decennial Supplement on Occupational Mortality (OPCS, 1986) makes possible a more comprehensive analysis of trends in inequalities of health for the country as a whole as well as by region. This allows the regional study to be put into perspective so that both research and policy priorities can be more readily identified. It also allows the nature of the nation's predicament over health to be clarified.

The problem is not just one of a North–South divide. Much of the recent public debate about health in Britain has fastened on to the differences between North and South. As the Health Education Council has most recently affirmed (HEC, 1987, p. 1), striking regional disparities in health can still be observed. 'From 1979–83 data, death rates were highest in Scotland, followed by the North and North West regions of England, and were lowest in the South East of England and East Anglia, confirming the long established North–South gradient.' However, these disparities are undercut by country-wide differences in the distribution of population by class and in the prevalence within classes of features of deprivation.

There is a national problem with regional overtones rather than a regional problem requiring isolated action. It is the purpose of this study to use available ward, regional and national statistics to map the dimensions of a deepening national problem. The exact definition of that problem requires a lot more work, but along with other recent studies, this book shows that the problem is becoming so important that it demands concerted national action to develop a better and more socially oriented programme of scientific research, to organise more effective health policies and to re-allocate resources.

The idea for this research arose in discussion with Mr Angus McNay, the Regional Statistician of the Northern Regional Health Authority in Newcastle. His enthusiastic support, and that of the Regional Health Authority General Manager, Mr Douglas Hague, has helped to turn an innovative research exercise into a substantial study.

A particular debt is due to the North Tyneside District Health Authority. This Authority has invited two of us (Peter Townsend and Peter Phillimore) to undertake research into inequalities in health in North Tyneside (the report of which will follow in 1988), and saw the value of a regional research project as well as a specialist study of their district. They gave every facility to enable a double programme of work to be mounted, and we are most grateful for their forbearance and support. Above all, we are deeply indebted to the late Dr Bryan Shaw and to Mr Tom Amos for their help in making our work possible, and to Mr Ray Layton for his constant advice and help.

For other support, advice, constructive criticism and active help we are also indebted to Assie Brower, David Byrne, Gill Durnell, John Fox, Nicky Hart, Belinda Maggs, Dr David Morris, Sarah Payne, Jacqui Perry, Sue Sadler, Alex Scott-Samuel, Melanie Smith, and Richard Wilkinson.

The views expressed in this book, and all remaining deficiencies are, of course, those of the authors alone.

Part One:

The Approach

1

Introduction: Aims, Concepts and Theories

The aim of this book is to examine and in part to explain current trends in inequalities of health in the United Kingdom, treating inequalities between the populations of the 678 wards making up the Northern Region of England as the primary subject-matter for detailed study. The book builds on two developing traditions of scientific work. One is the tradition of research describing, and seeking to explain, the widely varying health of people living in different areas. In Britain this has a long history. In the nineteenth century there were a large number of studies of public health, carefully measuring death rates from different diseases in particular localities (for example, Chadwick, 1842; Engels, 1958; and see accounts by historians — for example, Rosen, 1958; Lambert, 1961). That work gave impetus to the adoption of new public health policies because specific theories about area variations, like John Snow's proof that cholera was caused by impure water at the Broad Street Pump in 1849, could be put forward. In the depression years of the 1930s, such work on area inequalities in health came to play an important part in the nation's realisation of the need for a national health service (see, for example, Orr, 1936; M'Gonigle and Kirby, 1936; Titmuss, 1938). In the 1970s and 1980s work on area inequalities in health has burgeoned. (For the 1980s see OPCS, 1981; Howe, 1982; Bradshaw *et al.*, 1982; Irving and Rice, 1984; Fox *et al.*, 1984; Townsend *et al.*, 1984; Ashton, 1984; West of Scotland Politics of Health Group, 1984; Thunhurst, 1985a, b; Betts, 1985; Liverpool City Planning Department, 1986; Sheffield Health Authority, 1986). Such research was given fresh impetus by the Report of the Resource Allocation Working Party (DHSS, 1976). Area studies have posed questions simultaneously both about the objectives of health policies and the distribution of health

3

services, but they can scarcely be said to have begun to reflect a sophisticated mapping of social structure and organisation and hence properly to represent one alternative approach to scientific theory.

The other tradition of research has been of health in relation to social class. For Britain the work has covered most of the present century (Stevenson, 1928; Morris, 1975; Brotherston, 1976; Stacey, 1977; Hollingsworth, 1981; Hart, 1985) and has been a feature of the Registrar General's Decennial Supplements on Mortality (see for example OPCS, 1978 and 1986). In 1986 the theme has acquired a new impetus (Scott-Samuel, 1986), despite its depreciation in the latest of the Decennial Supplements (OPCS, 1986). There has also been a substantial number of studies in other countries, providing what one overseas observer has described as 'undisputed evidence of a strong negative association between socio-economic status and the probability of death' (Koskinen, 1985, p. 1). The results are well-attested and produce rather similar 'gradients' for different countries, whether socio-economic status or class is defined according to occupation (OPCS, 1978; Saull, 1983), education (Kitagawa and Hauser, 1973; Holme et al., 1980; Salonen, 1982; Saull, 1983), income (Rogers, 1979; Holme et al., 1980. Salonen, 1982; Wilkinson, 1986b) or some combination of these (Holme et al., 1980; Valkonen, 1982). The results apply to poorer countries and not only to European and North American countries (International Union for the Scientific Study of Population, 1984; United Nations, 1984. For North America, see, for example, Kosa et al., 1969; Antonovsky, 1972; and Kitagawa and Hauser, 1973). The differentials apply to nearly all causes of disease, though the gradient is much steeper for some diseases than others. For Britain in earlier years the gradient was found to be reversed for certain specific diseases, but these 'diseases of affluence' have now largely disappeared (Black Report, 1980, p. 70). The same has been demonstrated for Finland (Valkonen, 1982). The diseases which no longer provide the exceptions include non-valvular heart diseases (Marmot et al., 1978; Halliday and Anderson, 1979), peptic ulcer (Susser, 1962) and some malignant neoplasms (Logan, 1982).

Strenuous efforts have been and are being made to clarify and begin to explain the class gradient. One theme in research has been that upward and downward social mobility depends in part upon individual health. Ill people are presumed to descend and healthy people to ascend the occupational class scale. A further presumption is made that the perpetuation of inequalities of health between classes in Britain and in other countries is an artefact produced by the decline of unskilled and partly skilled classes at the foot of the social scale and the enlargement of the more prosperous skilled non-manual and manual classes. This theme has effectively been relegated to one of small importance by the reports on a longitudinal study by Fox and his colleagues (Fox and Goldblatt, 1982, Fox and Leon, 1985 and Fox *et al.*, 1985) and research into specific grades of a single occupation like that of Marmot and his colleagues (1978, 1985, 1986), and by detailed analytical reviews of the evidence.

Although there is evidence that social mobility is affected by ill-health and/or health potential, its contribution to observed class differences in health is probably always small in relation to the overall size of the mortality differentials. At older ages the condition may become almost insignificant (Wilkinson, 1986a, p. 16).

A very different theme is that, far from over-stating the effects upon health of differences in material living standards, the occupational class measure understates them. In particular, designation by occupational class may conceal a trend towards greater inequalities of health which may be attributed to greater inequalities in economic position or living standards. Firstly, with the decline of certain 'mass' occupations the variation in earnings within single occupations may now be quite marked. When taken in conjunction with the spread to home ownership (and the inheritance of housing) to manual families, the variation of living standards within occupations may be greater than in previous decades. Secondly, there is some variation in earnings for different occupations within a single occupational class. Thirdly, the risk of unemployment in the 1970s and 1980s introduces a further element of likely variation — certainly for manual groups — into occupational class as an indicator of living standards. Fourthly, the substantial importance for some groups of employer fringe benefits is not shared by other groups. Finally, the increased number and proportion of female partners holding paid jobs introduces a major element of potential variation into the living standards of families classified to the same occupational category.

As a consequence, it can be concluded that rankings by occupational class 'understate the true impact of socio-economic inequalities on health' (Wilkinson, 1986a, p. 17). Such a conclusion is supported by the analysis of mortality among civil servants by Marmot and his colleagues (1978, 1985). Two other general analyses of trends over several decades have shown that since 1951 the widening class differences in mortality, which were first properly described in the Black Report, are not a function of increased social mobility (Koskinen, 1985; Pamuk, 1985). One of these reviews has also shown that the use of different classifications in drawing up a ranking by occupational class and the changing numbers in occupations made little impact on the trends in mortality differentials (Pamuk, 1985). These comments suggest how difficult it is to move to an account of the methods and results of a particular piece of research, like the research on health in the Northern Region, without confronting the problems of concepts or definitions of health and those of the contextual theory which has necessarily to be adopted in any research. These will now be clarified.

1.1 CONCEPTS AND MODELS OF HEALTH

In all this work what must we understand by 'health'? In rich countries the concept of health has come under fierce scrutiny in the late twentieth century. Part of this has been due to a reaction against what has been perceived to be the dehumanising effects of medical ideology and technology when carried to extremes — as in features of the modern practice of chemotherapy, surgery and obstetrics (see, for example, Powles, 1973; Illich, 1975; Navarro, 1976; Ehrenreich, 1978; Stark, 1982). Medicine is felt to be too narrowly concerned with diseases, rather than with people. Another aspect of the scrutiny of health stems from a different reaction — against the artificial, clamorous and manufactured nature of modern urban life. The search for 'the good life' has become as important as the critique of medicine in changing attitudes to health and preparing people to consider different perspectives.

Scientifically there are two alternative modes of explanation. These were reviewed in the Black Report (1980, pp. 5–9). Firstly, there is the medical model. This is an engineering approach to health, built originally upon the Cartesian philosophy of the body conceived and controlled as a machine, and dealing essentially with the cure of diseases in individuals. We mean that the idea is carefully structured in terms of cure rather than prevention, disease rather than the promotion of health and welfare, and the examination and treatment of individual rather than of social conditions — whether of couples, friends, families, groups, communities or populations. The curious fact here is that in trying to escape the social and political controversies which are necessarily involved in, say, pursuing unremittingly

6

the reasons for differences in rates of mortality or morbidity between populations, or promoting the health and wellbeing of unemployed groups, or families living in poverty, or the population as a whole, the professional servant of medicine has accepted a circumspection of the scope of his or her work and a set of values which permits more than three-quarters of his or her potential scientific expertise and work to be drawn off and reconstituted as areas of political and bureaucratic responsibility. The restricted definition of responsibility for health has implications of which everyone should become aware. The development of knowledge to enlarge health is constrained. Some major social causes of ill-health and death are underestimated or ignored; and faith in the capacity of human beings to control the problems of life and liberate their potentialities is needlessly diminished.

The medical model is of course embodied in organisations and in the everyday analysis of fresh events. Ideas and meanings are not just disembodied abstractions; they are reflected in practice and structures. This means that priority is given in the allocation of resources to the prestigious departments of the practice of acute medicine, to specialised hospital treatment rather than general practice, and to casualty treatment instead of screening, prevention and health educa- tion. The use of the word 'ancillary' to denote someone whose work is defined to fit in with, but is clearly of lesser status than, that of medicine itself, is significant. Therefore the particular forms of the organisation and practice of health care in Britain and in other coun- tries reinforces the meaning of health central to the medical model. This is liable to be forgotten: even the critics of medicine will constantly be presented with examples of the re-affirmation of its prin- ciples which seem to deny any alternative.

Two qualifications have to be made to this summary representa- tion of the medical model. One is that it is not unambiguously consis- tent and clear-cut. The social is accommodated to the medicalised meaning of health. There are specialities which introduce the social aspects of health, like psychiatry, paediatrics and social medicine or epidemiology, but there is a degree of necessary intellectual sub- ordination or self-imposed submission. Thus, for example, epidemio- logy itself has generally been interpreted restrictedly as the study of the distribution of disease as the aggregate of individual phenomena (McMahon and Pugh, 1970; and see the critical discussion of Pater- son, 1982). In addition, some critics of medicine, who have argued that most of the decline in premature mortality in the nineteenth and twentieth centuries has been due to social changes like improvements in diet and living standards generally (in particular McKeown, 1976; but see also Winter, 1977 and 1981 for a valuable historical illustration), have sought more to call attention to the complementary features of an 'environmentalist' approach than to reconstitute medicine within an alternative model of health. The same is true of certain penetrating evaluations of medical care — using social factors, including class as a form of standardisation (for example Charlton *et al.*, 1983). They do not situate medicine as just one of the social institutions in an alternative model which seeks to explain the distribution of health. There are other ways in which medicine cannot be said to be 'monolithic'. There are forms of fringe medicine, like osteopathy, which are acceptable to many in the medical profession as well as to the public, as well as those forms which are unacceptable. Moreover, some conceptions of preventive action — albeit narrow or limited, and particularly when related to individual conditions or behaviour, such as check-ups or education about the risks of smoking or eating a diet heavy in cholesterol — are approved if not universally pursued.

Another qualification is equally important. Criticism of the medical 'model' which has developed must not be interpreted as cavalier rejection or disregard of certain benefits it has to offer. The challenge is in pursuing the larger questions about health to which medicine can offer only a partial or fragmented answer. Specialised features of medicine must therefore be incorporated into a larger model, parts of which are currently ill-developed. Certainly they are far less developed than some justly admired and honourable technologies and procedures of medicine. In contradistinction the social model of health takes as its basis the fact that human behaviour is ultimately social in its origin and determination, and depends upon social organisation and convention to encourage or restrain. People perform roles, have relationships and observe customs which are socially defined (including those which are made compulsory in an authoritarian state) and this provides the means both of identity and activity. This is not to say that people conform greyly to a uniform pattern: there are divergencies of age, background, environment and stage of family development which permit wide variation in personality and behaviour within any social structure, but the 'social' is what provides the necessary framework for observed health. It defines the pattern of daily life, diet, shelter, work and form of reproduction, upbringing and care; and it defines the variations between communities in adjoining areas as well as between cultures or nations. The vitality, endurance and freedom from disease, disability and stress — of individuals as much as of groups — can only be defined, explained and enhanced in that context.

The social approach to health is illustrated historically in the work of Virchow (1958) and Dubos (1959). Thus, in 1848 at the age of 27, Rudolf Virchow founded a journal entitled *Medizinische Reform*. He argued that poverty caused disease and that doctors had a duty to support social reforms to improve health. He believed that the treatment of individuals was only a small part of the practice of medicine and that the major part was the control of crowd diseases. This necessarily involved social and, if called for, even political measures. For him medicine was a social science. Dubos traced the origins and adoption of different ideas of health. He pointed out that before the late nineteenth century disease was generally regarded as resulting from a lack of harmony between the sick person and his or her environment, but with the work of Louis Pasteur, Robert Koch and their followers, medical opinion changed radically. They identified the virulent micro-organisms and through laboratory experiments they demonstrated that healthy animals could be made ill (see O'Brien (1982) for an account of changes of direction in the history of medicine).

The definition of health adopted upon the foundation of the World Health Organization is often quoted as a modern illustration of the social model of health as an alternative to the medical model. In fact it represents a rather lame compromise. The WHO defined health as 'a state of complete physical, mental and social well-being and not merely the absence of disease or infirmity'. (This theme was confirmed in the Alma-Ata declaration — Alma-Ata, 1978.) In fact, while emphasising positive in contrast to negative aspects of health, this definition conveys a curiously passive, steady-state idea of 'well-being' instead of one grounded in more active fulfilment — whether of productive work or useful and satisfying social roles and relationships. The definition implicitly favours an individual rather than a social orientation towards health, which may be said to perpetuate the wrong order of priorities in understanding and gaining control over the phenomenon. A more thoroughgoing social and dynamic conceptualisation has to be sought.

What are the implications of adopting a social model of health? Trained personnel would continue to work within the traditional practices of medicine but more of them would begin to work on prevention, on the early stages of disease and on recovery and rehabilitation. Of course it is not only 'health' but the social context of health which requires clarification to develop better theory to explain the distribution of health. We say 'social context' because the two traditions of research which we have identified — those of inequalities of health by area and by class — are imperfect representations of the population variations experienced in social structure and organisation and need to be better synthesised. Although some points will be discussed in ensuing chapters, certain introductory comments are required.

A 'social' model of health must reflect the pervasive characteristics of social institutions and state organisation. This means that society and not location must be treated as providing the causal mainspring of any local variations which may be observed in, say, health. Indeed some characteristics of 'location' are themselves socially rather than naturalistically derived — such as form of industry, enclosure and non-enclosure, waterways and roadways, afforestation or deforestation, vegetation and housing — and some of these features will ultimately be related to the history and present configuration of the ownership and price of land. So while there will be 'naturalistic' elements like climate or rock and land formation, many of them will have been adapted, reconstituted or overlaid by human use and will relate to, if not strictly conform with, social structure. The same points apply to the development of a concept of 'environment' to explain some of the effects of location upon health. Our necessary implication is that the *social* factors which themselves lie behind geographical, area or environmental variations in the distribution of health require identification.

A second necessary step is to accept that social class must not be regarded as just another social indicator, like employment status, tenure, race or overcrowding, but as *the* social concept which is fundamental to the explanation of the distribution of health — to which the listed indicators are secondarily related. In key respects this is a matter for scientific judgement (on the basis of empirical observation, experiment, statistical correlation, and theoretical consistency and integrity) and not mere ideology. As such, class must not be unnecessarily restricted to one aspect of social life, like occupation, but must be defined (operationally as well as in general principle) as a total reflection of differences in rank in economic and social position. This explains the Black Report's insistence on re-interpreting the usage of 'social' class in many commentaries on health as 'occupational' class (Black Report, 1980, p. 18).

The Registrar General has traditionally used an occupational classification as a basis for defining social class. A specific occupation may indeed denote, within narrow limits, what a person's earnings are likely to be, and therefore what income he or she and the household are likely to have, and the kind of home and the area they are likely to live in, as well as the amount of wealth they are likely to possess, the education they are likely to have had and even the kinds of customs and leisure activities they are likely to pursue. This is why in many studies of the past, occupational categorisation has 'worked' so well. It is because occupational status has borne an approximate correspondence, albeit a rough one, with class structure that explains its widespread use. However, that does not presuppose either that social class should be reduced to occupational status or that occupational status continues to be as good a proxy for social class as formerly. Both require contemporary attention. People's social class is fundamental to the opportunities in, and experience of, life. This can be demonstrated at each of the stages of pre-natal develop-ment, infancy, childhood, education, occupational career, marriage, child-rearing, post-family maturity and retirement.

The fact that it is more difficult to categorise people by social class than, say, by race or age does not mean that it is any less important or fundamental. Neither is the problem just one of methodological procedure — of finding how a population can be ranked in relation to an amalgam of resources, status, power situa-tion and disposition — it is in obtaining the necessary information in the first place; it is in appreciating that there are interests in society which are not particularly keen that such categorisations should be made, because questions would inevitably be raised about positions of wealth, power and privilege. Thus, it is difficult, for example, to take inherited wealth and the advantages of certain physical resources into account as factors in children's development and later recruitment to the grade as well as kind of jobs held. Perhaps the single most important component of 'class' which social scientists need to address is income — or a wider definition of income to include wealth and resources in kind, including fringe benefits (Townsend, 1979, Chapter 6). There is evidence that when successively more comprehensive and exact definitions of income are applied to a survey population, correlations with ill-health and disability are markedly more significant (ibid., p. 1176).

1.2 THE CONTEMPORARY CASE FOR A FRESH APPROACH

The need for a theory of health has become increasingly recognised in recent years and this study illustrates that need. Dissatisfaction with the cohesion of health care policies has been expressed independently, by bodies appointed by the British Government and by the DHSS itself. To different observers the failure to reduce inequalities in health, and the evident failure both to define and apply clear priorities which at a time of scarce resources utilise them economically, have become better recognised both by those in administrative control of services and by those studying or using them. Internationally there has been evidence of increasing percentages of Gross National Product being swallowed up by health care expenditure without any evident correlation between expenditure and health (Abel-Smith, 1967; Simanis, 1973; Abel-Smith, 1979; OECD, 1985). There have been calls for a more wide-ranging and fundamental approach to research (Alma-Ata, 1978), and research centres and institutes have been set up to proselytise an interdisciplinary approach (see the review by Stacey, 1980; also, Centre for Health Studies, Yale University, 1977).

In Britain the Department of Health has become sensitive to criticisms of its understanding as well as its direction of policy. The House of Commons Social Services Committee (House of Commons, 1980, paras 23–4) put the point comprehensively in its Third Report in 1980:

We would wish to emphasise, however, that the case for improving the Department's capacity to monitor the services for which it is accountable to Parliament does not rest solely on the need to assess the effects of expenditure changes on efficiency. The point has much wider implications. Our concern is to be able to assess the government's plans in terms of their effects on explicit policy aims. Our underlying question is: what is the NHS trying to do, and what is the relationship between expenditure plans and the government's policy objectives?

The Committee went on to deplore the lack of information about the likely effects of the Government's expenditure plans on its priorities and argues powerfully for a more effective system for both setting and monitoring priorities. In particular the Committee felt that inputs of resources explained little or nothing about the value of outputs of services to patients (House of Commons, 1980, paras 23–4). In a White Paper attempting to answer the criticisms, the Department admitted that information on final outputs — the benefit accruing to the individual or the community as a result of services provided — is more difficult to come by: mortality and morbidity rates partially fill this role, but even with these the full extent of the causal link between input and output is uncertain (UK Government, 1980, p. 8).

This book — especially its three-fold representation of 'health' in terms of measures of delayed development as well as of mortality and disablement — is intended to make some contribution to meeting criticisms of this kind.

How are more effective policies to be developed? — or, in the language of both the DHSS and its recent critics, how is the causal link between 'input' and 'output' to be supplied? Recent overseas and UK sources can be quoted to illustrate what work might be done. When making the case for a multi-disciplinary centre to study health at Yale University the proponents stated:

> By far the greatest proportion of resources devoted to recent research on ill-health by social, bio-medical, and public health scientists alike, has been allocated to the development of detection, diagnostic and curative techniques, the study of medical-care delivery, and the examination of preventive measures directed towards the alteration of individual behaviour (for example, Breslow and Wilner, 1977). While much research obviously remains to be done along these lines, there has been underestimation of both the social obstructions to health that lie beyond the competence of medicine alone to remedy, and the avenues to health open through social programmes far removed from medical care and from efforts to alter individual behaviour (Centre for Health Studies, Yale University, 1977, p. 2).

The group at Yale University went on to explain the alternative, or more comprehensive, approach. Because the kind of case made by the group is poorly understood and recognised, perhaps it deserves to be illustrated at some length. The connection between food and social institutions, for example, was carefully established.

> If dietary factors are implicated as proximate risks for colon cancer or for heart disease, they must be understood in combination with other social factors, for example, perhaps, a life-style requiring quick, high energy foods, the vulnerability of

13

consumers to food advertising, the use of chemical feeds for market livestock, the use of chemical additives in foods, the availability of only certain types of foods in the market place, and the structure of the . . . food industry (ibid, p. 8).

All were clearly implicated not only in understanding cause, but also in developing policy.

Health differences between areas clearly constitute something which goes beyond individual self-management and physiological functioning, but which also goes beyond mere matters of soil and climate.

The problems of occupational or public exposure to such risks as lead, asbestos, noise or vinyl chloride, for instance, are issues far beyond the pale of biomedical competence or individual prudence, and touch on such basic social issues as the organisation of factory labour, the management of industry, and the role of unions and collective bargaining. And yet policy to curb such exposures might have a beneficient impact on health far greater than the combined impacts of improved treatment or efforts to alter individual behaviour (ibid, p. 8).

One interesting idea in this social model of health was to track elements harmful to individuals to their social sources. Thus, research might

attempt to map the distribution and transmission of potentially dangerous substances, for example, certain carcinogens, in the economy. This could be accomplished with an eye to appropriate interventions. Such an effort would begin by assembling data on known carcinogenic content and effluents by product and process. Utilising input-output techniques, the direct and indirect flows of carcinogens through the economy would be traced, with attribution of carcinogen production to various final products and types of final demand (ibid, p. 9).

In Britain the recent work of environmental chemists provides a fine example. The zinc deficiency in modern diets, argued in some research to be related to conditions such as anorexia nervosa, has been attributed to three modern agricultural practices:

(1) the use of phosphate fertilisers which render zinc less readily taken up by growing plants;

(2) the failure to maintain the organic content of many soils; and
(3) the failure to re-cycle zinc (as well as other nutritionally essential trace elements) to soils. (Bryce-Smith, 1986, p. 118.)

The exact pattern of relationships remains to be confirmed. The toxic effects of even low levels of lead have also been shown to have more serious effects than was formerly believed. Elevated traces of lead and cadmium and zinc deficiency seems to be correlated with serious malformation, poor foetal development and low birthweight.

Of all environmental pollutants so far identified, the neurotoxin lead is evidently the most serious and widespread in its subtle and insidious impact on man. There now appears to be no observable threshold for its toxic effects on the development and function of the child's brain . . . adverse mental effects . . . and blood pressure (Bryce-Smith, 1986, pp. 118–22).

One of the social institutions relatively neglected in developing a theory of health is the family. Those setting up the centre at Yale asked, for example,

To what extent does family solidarity, other group affliction, or social cohesion modify the effects on physical health (not just mental health) of various kinds of occupational stress? What are the mechanisms that lead, from the instability of family and marriage, as well as from changed family functions, to ill-health? . . . What is the relationship, if any, of various public policies on the ability of family solidarity to mediate stress? (Centre for Health Studies, Yale University, 1977, pp. 10–11)

Even more instructive is to examine the implications for health in a wide set of national policies not expressly directed at health. They may

nonetheless, have enormous (sometimes adverse) impact on health. Those that are not explicitly aimed at health might include policies on, for example, energy, transit and highways, industrial technologies, industrial location, corporate autonomy, unemployment, social security, education, occupational training, race discrimination, housing and income distribution. As a nation [the reference being to the United States] we have ignored the health consequences of these policies (ibid. pp. 8, 9 and 12).

These quotations help to set out the powerful case which exists for a re-statement of health theory.

In the United Kingdom, perhaps the best illustration of this approach is the Report of the Working Group on Inequalities in Health, under the chairmanship of Sir Douglas Black (frequently referred to as the Black Report). The Working Group devoted a chapter of its 1980 report to the need for additional information and research for the development of better theory. This immediately followed its analysis of the causes of inequalities in health. The Working Group accepted that cultural and genetic factors played an important role but concluded that 'material deprivation' was the predominant factor in explaining inequalities. Too little, however, was known about its form and impact and the Working Group therefore proposed that there were two very important means of developing our knowledge. One was through the longitudinal approach, and the three longitudinal health surveys provide examples (1946, 1958 and 1970 cohorts — see for example Douglas, 1951; Douglas and Walker, 1966; Davie et al., 1972; Colley et al., 1973; Douglas and Gear, 1976; Wadsworth and Morris, 1978; Butler, 1977; Butler and Osborne, 1985). Another approach using the longitudinal method is provided by following up a small percentage of census data (see, for example, Fox and Leon, 1985).

The other means of developing knowledge recommended in the Black Report was

> the way in which economic, social and environmental variables interact within small geographical areas. Such a study would be limited to a small number of such areas, selected on the basis of social condition or health data. It would involve collection of detailed economic, social, environmental and occupational data, as well as data on the health, ill-health and mortality of the population. Such a study, we believe, would also permit far more detailed appreciation of the health effects of social and economic policies (without the need to assume the independence of such policies) than is possible from aggregate level data (Black Report, 1980, p. 223).

The Working Group also called for the development of indicators of area social conditions and health — especially for use in resource allocation, and for further research into health hazards in relation to occupational conditions and work. These lend themselves to research in small areas and might be said to reinforce the case for choosing to undertake a study of the interaction of social factors implicated in ill-health. In particular, the Working Group called for further work to be undertaken into the use of occupational class as an indicator: it called both for the development of a composite indicator of family class (amalgamating the occupations of husband, wife and their respective fathers) and research to distinguish the direct and indirect association between occupation and health. Too little was known about the conditions and amenities of work, as distinct from the specific hazards of certain industrial conditions (for a detailed review of one aspect of the relationship between occupations and health, see Harrington, 1978).

What are the administrative and political implications of adopting a social model of health? Trained personnel would continue to work within the traditional practices of medicine but more of them would begin to work on prevention, the early stages of disease, and recovery and rehabilitation. More emphasis would necessarily be given to relief from pain, discomfort, stress and boredom, but also to education for health and participation in local and national measures to deal with common family and community problems and promote new modes of organisation. A 'health' policy would represent a version of existing housing, environmental health, safety at work, anti-pollution and public protection services in which priorities were more clearly established. Health personnel would work in a greater variety of social contexts. At the present time neither local nor national policies constitute concerted strategies which are related to operational information about the health of the population and which seek to co-ordinate the work of different administrative departments. Whether that can be achieved will depend on the capacity of the social and medical sciences to provide a social model of health to transform the nature of health care much as Newton and his successors transformed the nature of physics in the eighteenth century.

2

The Northern Region and the
North–South Divide

This chapter introduces the chief case-study on which the analysis in this book is based. Later chapters (9 and 10) examine evidence nationally and for other regions more closely. Throughout this century the North of England has experienced high mortality in comparison with the country as a whole. This study is not the first to document the existence of inequalities of health within the towns and cities of the North and to pick out the Region's problems. Fifty years ago the Medical Officer of Health for Stockton-on-Tees, G.C.M. M'Gonigle, and his sanitary inspector, J. Kirby, published *Poverty and public health* (1936).

M'Gonigle used 1931 Census data and mortality data for the period 1928–32, showing, for example, that while Stockton as a whole had an age-standardised quinquennial death rate of 12.07 per thousand, the rate in the Mount Pleasant area was 33.55 and the rate in the Riverside area was 22.78 (ibid., 1936, p. 122). He further described the difference in death rates between employed and unemployed people living in the same area of Stockton. Both rates were higher than the national rate, but the rate for the unemployed was almost 30 per cent higher than that for the employed (ibid., 1936, p. 268). He then took all 777 families and ranked them in groups according to income level, calculating the death rate for each group. The results showed that there was 'a regular decline in death-rate with regular increase in income level' (ibid., 1936, p. 273).

M'Gonigle also reported 'A Newcastle investigation', undertaken by Dr J.C. Spence, into the health and nutrition of certain children in the city. Two groups of children were clinically examined: 125 'city children', the parents of 105 of whom were then unemployed; and 124 children of 'better class families', the 'professional families class'. Spence showed that the 'professional class' children were,

18

age for age, both heavier and taller than the 'city children' (ibid., 1936, p. 134). There was also a difference in the number of anaemic children in each group and the records made of each child's various illnesses showed that 'infections and other diseases were more frequent and occurred at an earlier age in the city group than in the professional families group' (ibid., 1936, p. 138). Spence had concluded that the main factors contributing to physical ill-health were poor housing conditions, which explained widespread infectious diseases among young children, and unsatisfactory diet, which frustrated recovery from illness. One general aim of this study is to re-open some of these lines of enquiry in relation to present health patterns, and to provide a basis for more detailed research into variations in health.

2.1 POPULATION AND ECONOMY

An understanding of the unequal distribution of health in the North of England depends first on a knowledge of population and ecology. Cleveland, Cumbria, Durham, Northumberland, and Tyne and Wear, the five most northerly counties of England, form an extremely diverse region. The population of 3.1 million (OPCS, mid-1984 estimate) is concentrated in the east, to such an extent that around three-quarters live within 25 miles of the east coast (Smail, 1985, p. 1), predominantly close to the conurbations of Tyneside, Wearside and Teesside. By contrast, the northern end of the Pennine chain, the Cheviot Hills, and the hills of the Lake District, mean that Northumberland, Cumbria and the western part of Durham have low population densities: indeed, at 60 people per square kilometre, Northumberland is the most sparsely populated county in England (Central Statistical Office, 1985). On a small scale, however, the west coast mirrors the east, with the majority of the Cumbrian population living in the coastal strip between Carlisle and Barrow.

Economically, a long history of decline in the traditional heavy industries of coal-mining, steel production, ship-building and heavy engineering, the inability of new sources of employment to offset losses in the old, and consequent high levels of unemployment, have all been characteristic of the Northern Region for several decades. The present recession during the late 1970s and 1980s, however, has magnified enormously the pressures on this historically vulnerable regional economy, as all the traditional industries, coupled this time with the massive chemical industry on Teesside, have contracted even further. One outcome has been that today around 60 per cent of employees work in the service sector, whilst just over one-quarter are employed in all manufacturing industries. The trend is visible even over as short a period as seven years, for in 1977 one-half of the workforce was employed in the service sector, with over one-third in manufacturing (Smail, 1985, p. 1). It is also the case that the Northern Region has experienced the highest unemployment rate of all regions in mainland Britain throughout the last 20 years, with the highest regional percentage of long-term unemployment (more than 26 weeks). The North is the only region to have a smaller civilian working population in 1985 than in 1975 (Central Statistical Office, 1986). As will be seen later, unemployment is predictably greatest in the major urban centres of the north-east (Tyneside, Sunderland, Hartlepool and Teesside) in much of Durham (nowhere more so than in Consett), and in the towns of the West Cumbrian coastal strip. However, rural areas have not escaped either, especially in the upland areas of the northern Pennines. In these areas, moreover, 'real' levels of unemployment are often disguised by the young moving away in search of work.

This picture of the Northern Region, which will be familiar to many people, has its counterpart when we turn to health in the Region — except that in this case the details are not widely known: for not only does the North have a depressed economy, by comparison with nearly all other regions in the country[1] [footnotes in this book are listed on p. 159]; it also experiences worse health, as measured through official statistics. The most commonly used measure of a population's health for many years has been the mortality rate (see the Black Report, 1980). On this criterion, the North invariably fares badly. Only the North-West of the English Standard Regions experiences overall mortality as high as the North at the present time, and these two have consistently had the highest death rates in England throughout the post-war era (OPCS Area Mortality Statistics, DH5, 1981–3; OPCS Area Mortality Decennial Supplement, 1969–73). Comparing the recently abolished metropolitan counties of England also shows that mortality for men in Tyne and Wear has been as high if not higher than anywhere else during the last decade, although women's mortality has generally been higher in Merseyside and Greater Manchester, at least in recent years (ibid.).

In addition to the North and North-West, Scotland, Wales and Northern Ireland also suffer from high mortality; and just how high these death rates are in relation to many European countries can be

Table 2.1: Age standardised mortality from all causes in 1980

RATES PER 100,000 POPULATION AGED 40–69 YEARS

TOTAL POPULATION (MEN AND WOMEN) MILLIONS		Men	Women		TOTAL POPULATION (MEN AND WOMEN) MILLIONS
10.7	Hungary	1842	917	Hungary	10.7
15.3	Czechoslovakia	1702	866	SCOTLAND	5.0
35.6	Poland	1701	840	Romania	22.2
5.0	SCOTLAND	1542	802	NORTHERN IRELAND	1.5
4.8	Finland	1504	797	NORTHERN REGION	3.1
3.1	NORTHERN REGION	1496	779	Ireland	3.4
1.5	NORTHERN IRELAND	1492	776	Czechoslovakia	15.3
22.2	Romania	1464	763	New Zealand	3.1
22.3	Yugoslavia	1385	746	Poland	35.6
8.8	Bulgaria	1363	746	Yugoslavia	22.3
3.4	Ireland	1360	736	Bulgaria	8.8
7.5	Austria	1342	692	Denmark	5.1
9.8	Belgium	1322	687	ENGLAND AND WALES	49.6
227.7	USA	1296	685	Israel	3.9
61.5	West Germany	1270	672	USA	227.7
49.6	ENGLAND AND WALES	1267	631	Austria	7.5
3.1	New Zealand	1253	622	SOUTH EAST REGION	17.0
53.7	France	1223	620	Belgium	9.8
5.1	Denmark	1214	607	West Germany	61.5
57.0	Italy	1203	582	Australia	14.7
14.7	Australia	1194	581	Canada	24.0
24.0	Canada	1159	546	Finland	4.8
17.0	SOUTH EAST REGION	1141	544	Italy	57.0
14.1	Netherlands	1078	516	Sweden	8.3
4.1	Norway	1076	496	France	53.7
6.4	Switzerland	1021	496	Netherlands	14.1
8.3	Sweden	1014	487	Switzerland	6.4
3.9	Israel	1012	480	Norway	4.1
116.8	Japan	905	470	Japan	116.8

Sources: Uemura & Pisa (1985); and *UN Statistical Yearbook 1982.*

Table 2.2: The regional distribution of sickness and invalidity in Britain

% all persons aged 16+ permanently sick, 1981		Spells of certified incapacity due to sickness and invalidity, 1982–3: per 100 Men		per 100 Women	
1.		2.		3.	
1. Wales	3.12	Wales	35.3	North-West	42.7
2. NORTH	2.53	NORTH	33.1	Wales	41.0
3. North-West	2.22	North-West	32.0	Scotland	40.4
4. Scotland	2.04	Scotland	31.1	Gtr. London	34.8
5. Yorks-Humber	2.00	Yorks-Humber	30.4	Yorks-Humber	32.8
6. W. Midlands	1.70	E. Midlands	27.3	NORTH	32.5
7. South-West	1.65	W. Midlands	22.9	E. Midlands	29.9
8. E. Midlands	1.61	Gtr. London	21.9	South-East	28.4
9. Gtr. London	1.49	South-West	21.4	South-West	27.5
10. East Anglia	1.33	South-East	20.1	W. Midlands	27.4
11. South-East	1.24	East Anglia	19.2	East Anglia	25.0
BRITAIN	1.80		26.0		33.3
Ratio of North to best region	2.0		1.7		1.3

Sources: Col. 1: OPCS, 1981 Census. Cols 2 and 3: *Social Security Statistics*, 1984 (DHSS); and OPCS, 1981 Census.
Notes: Cols 2 and 3: Figures for Scotland and Wales are based on the population covered by National Insurance. Such data are not produced for the English regions. As a close approximation, the economically active population at the 1981 Census (aged 16+) has been taken, and then adjusted by the factor necessary to reduce the England economically active total in 1981 to the England insured population total in 1982–3. This means the relative rank of the regions is based on the economically active population, but the figures allow a more accurate reflection of female in relation to male sickness patterns. South-East denotes the standard region of this name excluding Greater London.

shown from the international comparisons which are available. Table 2.1 gives figures for a range of industrialised countries, and also for the Northern and South-Eastern Regions of England. These two Regions are picked out because of current interest in the North–South debate. The rate in the North shown in the table is 31 per cent higher than for the South-East. Other countries' regions are not separately identified, but it should be remembered that, with a population of more than three million, the Northern Region is as large as, or not much smaller than, several central and northern European countries. If the lowest ranking European country is used as a standard (Sweden in the case of men, Norway in the case of women), then the Northern Region has an 'excess' male death rate of 48 per cent in the 40–69 age range, and an 'excess' female rate of 66 per cent. If we turn from death to sickness and incapacity a similar picture also emerges. Measuring ill-health poses problems which do not arise with mortality (see below, section 3.1). Even so, the evidence presented in Table 2.2 suggests that the Northern Region has among the highest levels of sickness in the country, rivalled only by Wales, Scotland and the North-West Region. The latest OPCS Report (1986) further confirms its relative disadvantages, as we shall explore in Chapter 10.

Now the main purpose of the present study is to highlight the considerable difference in health *within* the North, at the smallest and most local level feasible for analysis — namely, the local authority ward level. However, a major reason for doing so is the fact that this Region as a whole experiences such poor health, in relation to most parts of the country. The inequalities in health within the North are more than simply the regional reflection of the national inequalities documented in the Black Report (1980): for the Northern Region is not a microcosm of the country as a whole, but one of its most deprived constituent parts — in economic and in health terms. This study is therefore concerned with health inequalities within an area identified as being biased towards the worse end of the spectrum of health in this country.

If differences in health are apparent enough at regional level, this is even more true at Health or Local Government District level. Table 2.3, based on mortality data, offers an initial indication of the inequality which exists between districts within the North, but also of how skewed the distribution is towards the worse end of the national health spectrum. The worst-placed districts in the North, with mortality between 20 and 25 per cent above the national average, contrast markedly with those others, overwhelmingly rural, where mortality is better than the national average. However, the latter are few, and account for only a small part of the North's population.

Along with Scotland, the West Midlands and the North-West, the North stands out among the regions of Britain which have the widest inequalities of health between classes within their boundaries. This is illustrated by the wide differences between non-manual and manual occupational classes in their standardised mortality ratios. In the North the rate for male manual workers as a whole is nearly half as much again as for non-manual workers (Table 2.4).

The really striking feature which emerges from this chapter is the

Table 2.3: Regional and district mortality: the Northern Region compared with the South-East and South-West Regions

	1981	1982	1983
Mortality ratios: NORTH SOUTH-EAST SOUTH-WEST	113 93 91	112 94 92	111 93 92
L.G. Districts in North among 20 with highest mortality in England and Wales (Mortality ratios in parentheses)	Hartlepool (126) Derwentside Middlesbrough Copeland Easington Wear Valley Chester-le-Street Langbaurgh (119)	Hartlepool (124) Middlesbrough Copeland Easington Gateshead Stockton Wear Valley Berwick (120)	Copeland (122) Sedgefield Middlesbrough Easington Gateshead (117)
No. of districts in S.E. and and S.W. in highest 20	0	1	0
Districts in North among 20 in England and Wales with lowest mortality	0	0	0
Best Northern district	Castle Morpeth (91)	South Lakeland (93)	Teesdale (72)
No. of districts in S.E. and S.W. among 20 in England and Wales with lowest mortality	16	14	18

Source: OPCS Local Authority Vital Statistics, 1981, 1982, 1983.
Notes: Data for 1981 and 1982 are based on Adjusted Mortality Ratios (AMRs); 1983 data on Standardised Mortality Ratios (SMRs), following a change by OPCS (see Glossary). Castle Morpeth has been excluded from the 1983 list of high mortality districts, in line with the OPCS recommendations on the interpretation of district SMRs (see Bulusu, 1985). The high mortality bloc contains 20, 24 and 21 districts; the low mortality bloc 20, 19 and 22 in the three selected years.

Table 2.4: SMRs for all causes 1979–80, 1982–3 for manual and non-manual occupations by region, men aged 20–64. Ranking of regions by manual SMR/non-manual SMR

Standard region/country	Ratio (1):(2)	Non-manual (1)[a]	Manual (2)[a]
Scotland	1.56	93.3	145.8
North	1.48	88.5	131.1
West Midlands	1.48	79.6	118.0
North-West	1.47	89.8	131.8
Wales	1.42	84.4	120.2
South-East	1.42	72.7	103.4
Yorkshire and Humberside	1.37	85.3	117.1
South-West	1.36	73.3	99.5
East Midlands	1.31	80.0	104.8
East Anglia	1.25	68.9	85.8
Great Britain	1.46	79.6	116.1

Note: a. SMR for all men in Great Britain in 1979–80, 1982–3 is 100.
Source: OPCS (1986) *1979–80, 1982–83, Occupational Mortality*, HMSO, London, Microfiche tables GD38.

extreme nature of the contrast between districts in the North, on the one hand, and in the two southern regions, the South-East and South-West, on the other. The only district in the two southern regions which ranks on a par with the worst Northern districts is Tower Hamlets in London; and with this single exception, those southern districts with the highest mortality (almost all in London) correspond to districts which in the North are close to the middle of the regional distribution.

2.2 NORTH AND SOUTH: CHANGES IN 50 YEARS

How can the changes in health in different regions of the UK be captured? With the decline in mortality during the twentieth century, there has been a large shift in the proportions of deaths occurring at different ages. Life expectation has risen through the combination of a dramatic fall in the numbers of people dying in infancy and childhood, and a more gradual decline in death rates at other ages. In 1931, 58 per cent of male deaths and 50 per cent of female deaths in England and Wales occurred before the age of 65; by 1983 the equivalent figures were 27 per cent and 16 per cent respectively.

We can compare these national trends in mortality with present-day area variations within Britain. There are big differences in

Figure 2.1: The distribution by age of all deaths under 75 years

0–14	15–44	45–64	65–74	
21	22	56	76	= 175

ENGLAND AND WALES 1936–8

| 8 | 11 | 47 | 70 | = 136 |

ENGLAND AND WALES 1950–2

| 3 | 7 | 36 | 54 | = 100 |

ENGLAND AND WALES 1981–3

| 4 | 7 | 48 | 66 | = 125 |

MIDDLESBROUGH DISTRICT 1981–3

| 3 | 5 | 29 | 46 | = 83 |

GUILDFORD DISTRICT 1981–3

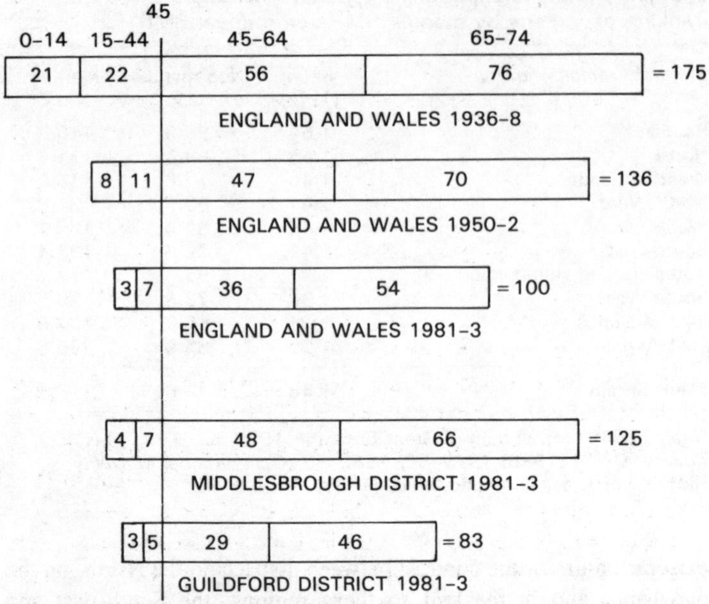

Note: England and Wales 1981–3 = 100

health experience between populations. This can also be interpreted in terms of some populations still being locked into the health experience of earlier decades. Figure 2.1 compares the distribution by age at death of all deaths under 75 years for England and Wales at three different periods over the last 50 years (1936–8, 1950–2 and 1981–3). These in turn are compared with the distributions for one northern district, Middlesbrough, and one southern district, Guildford, in 1981–3 (all populations have been standardised to England and Wales, 1981). The purpose is to highlight how much some populations have still to catch up with national improvements. The format shows both the relative proportions of deaths in each of four age bands (0–14, 15–44, 45–64 and 65–74), and also absolute levels of mortality. Middlesbrough and Guildford have been chosen as representative of the two extremes of mortality in England and Wales at the present time, Middlesbrough featuring among the 20 local government districts with the highest overall mortality in England and Wales for 1981, 1982 and 1983; whereas Guildford features among the 20 local authorities with the lowest mortality in England and Wales for two of these three years.

26

In Figure 2.1, England and Wales mortality between 1981 and 1983 is taken as the standard and for every one hundred deaths under the age of 75, the number occurring at different ages is illustrated. In comparison, if Middlesbrough's age-specific death rates occurred nationally 125 deaths, not 100 deaths, would be experienced, with the greatest percentage increase over the national rate being in the 45–64 range; whereas if Guildford's death rates applied nationally, only 83 deaths would occur, with the largest decrease being in the 45–64 range. By going on to place national data from the late 1930s and early 1950s alongside current figures, present trends can be put into historical perspective. One lesson to be drawn is that, whilst inequalities certainly persist today under 45 (as we will show in the more fine-grained analysis of the North later in this study), they are slight when set alongside the massive improvement since the years before and after the Second World War. Although Middlesbrough is currently an area of high mortality, its mortality experience at ages under 45 is closer to an area like Guildford than to the experience of the country as a whole 30 or 45 years previously.

The reverse is the case when we look at the next age band, from 45–64. This is the range which provides the widest current inequalities in mortality between one area and another, and, because of the numbers of deaths involved, contributes most to these differentials. In contrast with the under-45s, in areas like Middlesbrough, mortality between 45 and 64 is directly comparable with the national experience of the early 1950s, and no great improvement on the late 1930s. It is not hard to envisage that at the local level, these historical parallels would be even more pronounced where recent mortality is especially high. It is thus in deaths in the 20-year period from the mid-40s to the mid-60s of the age span that areas of high mortality, at least in the North, most clearly lag behind the country as a whole.

2.3 NORTH AND SOUTH: THE GAP TODAY

The sharp differences in mortality between districts in the North like Middlesbrough, and those in the South, like Guildford, can also be matched in indicators of living standards. Thus, in October 1986, the rate of unemployment in Middlesbrough was, according to the Department of Employment, 25.9 per cent (or, according to the Unemployment Unit, 30.5 per cent), compared with 4.2 per cent in Guildford (or 4.9 per cent). (*Unemployment Bulletin*, Winter 1986,

Table 2.5: North and South: some indicators of living standards

Indicator	North	South-East	Ratio of North to South-East	Rank position of North (9 regions of England & Wales)
Unemployment rate, 1985 (per cent)	18.9	9.9	1.9	highest
Annual redundancies per 1,000 employees (1982–5)	26	7	3.7	highest
Households with no car (per cent)	48.3	35.9	1.3	highest
Households with no telephone (per cent)	31.0	15.5	2.0	highest
Households with no central heating (per cent)	31.1	29.1	1.1	7th highest
Households not owner-occupied (per cent)	46	37	1.24	highest
Pupils taking free school meals (per cent)	25.4	12.2	2.1	highest
16 year-olds leaving full-time education (per cent)	79.5	69.8	1.14	highest
Average weekly household income (1983)	£163.8	£230.7	0.71	lowest
GDP per head (1984)	£4,154	£5,402	0.77	3rd lowest
Personal disposable income per head (1984)	£3,512	£4,456	0.79	3rd lowest
Amount per head spent in region on supplementary benefit (1983–4)	£123.5	£92.9	1.33	highest
Weekly expenditure of household on food	£28.0	£32.9	0.85	lowest
Weekly expenditure of household on alcohol	£7.6	£7.5	1.01	highest
Weekly expenditure of household on tobacco	£5.0	£3.8	1.32	highest
Stillbirth rate (1984)	6.3	5.3	1.19	highest
Perinatal mortality rate (1984)	11.0	9.3	1.18	3rd highest
Infant mortality rate (1984)	9.4	9.0	1.04	3rd highest
SMR (1984)	112	92	1.22	highest
Births under 2500 gm (1984)	7.1	6.9	1.03	4th highest
Adults perm. sick or disabled (per cent)	2.5	1.3	1.9	highest

Sources: Central Statistical Office, *Regional Trends*, 21, 1986, HMSO, London; OPCS, *1981 Census, National Report*; OPCS Population and Vital Statistics Series Vs. No. 11.

pp. 19–20). Table 2.5 compares some general indicators of standards of living in the North and the South-East. On a number of criteria of material deprivation, the North ranks worst among the regions of England and Wales and is markedly worse placed than the South-East. For several years the North has had much the highest rate of redundancies. One of the most significant differences is in personal disposable income — that is, income after deductions for tax and national insurance contributions. Earnings are lower and more people depend on supplementary benefit. Relative personal disposable income per head fell from 96 per cent of the national average in 1982 to only 90 per cent in 1984. During the ten years to 1984 there was a similar decline in relative GDP per head. 'The North was the only region of the United Kingdom in which the civilian working population (which includes the unemployed) was smaller in 1985 than it had been in 1975' (Central Statistical Office, 1986, p. 11).

In sum, this chapter has shown that the North has a long history of deprivation and high mortality. Despite post-war improvements at the younger ages in mortality, improvements at the older ages have been small in recent decades. The health of the North stands poor comparison, not only with the rest of England and Wales, but with nearly all major regions of Europe. A matter of deep concern is the worsening of some economic indicators relative to the average in Britain.

3

Indicators of Health and Deprivation

A concept with as many elements of meaning as the concept of 'health' — health as the absence of disease; health as freedom from pain, discomfort or sickness; health as fitness or mobility; health as mental and physical well-being; health as full membership of society, with participation in a range of roles — is too subtle and all-embracing to be measured easily. Suitable statistical indicators are few, and in any case these only cover certain dimensions of health, leaving many others beyond the reach of measurement — or at least, measurement on a national or regional basis.

3.1 THE CONSTRUCTION OF A MEASURE OF HEALTH

In this study, we have relied upon the following kinds of health data, all of which cover the whole population, a prerequisite for a study of small areas: death registration data, from which mortality indicators can be derived, chiefly but not exclusively in the form of standardised mortality ratios (SMRs — see Glossary, p. 161); data on births, from which birthweight indicators can be constructed; and data on rates of permanent sickness or disability. No other health information exists at present which covers the whole of the population and can be analysed at a level as localised as the ward. In the next chapter we present the evidence of the distribution of ill-health in the North. To do this we have relied on three specific measures of health, namely, premature mortality, permanent sickness and disablement and delayed development in infancy. These form the foundations of our analysis. These measures are:

(1) *Premature mortality.* Standardised Mortality Ratios for persons

(i.e. both sexes together) under 65 years (0–64) based on deaths over three years, 1981–3.
(2) *Permanent sickness and disablement.* The proportion of all residents in private households aged 16 and over who classed themselves as permanently sick or disabled at the 1981 Census.
(3) *Low birthweight and delayed development.* The proportion of live births below 2,800 gm, (6 lbs 2.75 ozs) based on births over three years, 1982–4.

Further information on data sources and definitions will be found in Appendix 1. In addition, we have combined these three individual measures to form an 'Overall Health Index', assigning equal weight to each of the three components. These are not the sole health indicators used in this study, but they are the primary ones. In presenting the evidence on mortality, in particular, a variety of indicators will be used at different points. The three distinct dimensions of health set out above — namely, mortality, morbidity (chronic sickness and disablement), and low birthweight and delayed infant development — represent contemporary interpretations of health. Considering how few health statistics are available for the illustration of differences between areas, it is not surprising that these or similar measures crop up in several other studies (Scott-Samuel, 1984; Townsend *et al.*, 1984; Hume and Womersley, 1985; Leavey and Wood, 1985). To our knowledge, this is the first study to combine these particular measures in an overall index. Some comment on the actual specification of the variables is now necessary.

On mortality, 65 has been taken as the upper age limit in order to identify unambiguously what is by common consent premature mortality. People over this age are also difficult to classify on existing scales of inequality, because occupational designations are less reliable as a guide to social position and alternative information is not available (Townsend and Davidson, 1982, p. 56). Initially we considered separating an adult mortality variable (15–64) from an infant or infant and childhood one (0–1 or 0–14), but, given the small numbers of infant and child deaths in wards, and the effect on the rate in a small ward of a variation of only a couple of deaths, it seemed less misleading to adopt a single variable covering the first 65 years of life. In doing so, the possibility of distinguishing differences in patterns of infant and child mortality has been reluctantly set aside. Any reliable study of those patterns for small areas in Britain will depend on obtaining data for a longer span of years.

31

Inevitably the aggregation of deaths between 0 and 64 will be dominated by the relatively large number of deaths in the 20 years leading up to 65. However, where possible, we have looked at smaller age-groups within this aggregation in this study.

The importance of the start of life is, however, covered in our data by the choice of birthweight as a key indicator. This variable helps to balance the other two variables, which are heavily influenced by the health of the middle-aged and older age-groups. It is a sensitive measure of infant development (although it may not always denote delayed development) and also carries implications for maternal health. In recent OPCS and other studies a weight of under 2,500 gm has been taken as defining low birthweight. Although, for comparison with other work, some information on births under 2,500 gm is presented below, the higher weight of 2,800 gm has been preferred as the dividing line in this study. This is in order to include a higher proportion of births and to lessen the chance of anomalies affecting the ward ranking by virtue of small numbers in the 'tail' of many distributions. This is in line with the Bristol study by Townsend *et al.* (1984).

A recurrent source of frustration in epidemiological research has been the lack of measures of sickness or disability covering the whole population. Morbidity data are notoriously sparse. In 1980, Brennan and Clare pointed out the potential value of the sickness data in the Census; and since then a number of studies have used the proportion of permanently sick or disabled at the Census (i.e. Scott-Samuel, 1984; Leavey and Wood, 1985). However, such information is only available every ten years and cannot be analysed by age or class. Moreover, it relates to an economic condition (the cause of economic inactivity), which makes it suspect for differentiating male and female patterns, and is not strictly speaking a measure of morbidity. Whereas births and deaths are registered and undisputed events, information on permanent sickness and disablement is based on self-reporting alone.

One point to acknowledge about these three indicators is that, whilst SMRs give a clear and strong representation of an area's experience of mortality, the permanent sickness and low birthweight indicators provide somewhat less direct representations of the aspects of health which they are intended to reflect: levels of adult chronic sickness and disablement, and potential child development and maternal health. Yet if each of these indicators is useful in its own right, what advantage is there in combining them? In our view, there are good reasons favouring the use of a summary variable: it allows us to weigh up the relative extent of a ward's premature mortality, chronic sickness and low birthweight, in order to reach an overall assessment of its position in health terms. This summary is admittedly fairly approximate, but it does cover three key dimensions of health, and we believe it also has implications for social policy as one attempt to go beyond excessive reliance on mortality data in the assessment of an area's health. Moreover, all we are doing is presenting a sociologicallly reasoned version of a process we all undertake in daily life: for in reality, people do not generally evaluate localities as more or less desirable or satisfactory just on a series of separate yardsticks; they also try to reach an overall judgement by weighing up the various criteria together.

There are also other considerations. The larger the number of health-related events or experiences covered in an indicator, the more we can overcome the potential difficulty with a ward-level analysis of working with small populations. The smaller the ward, of course, the more this applies: for instance, in a hypothetical medium-sized ward there might be 80 deaths over three years among people under 65. By putting these alongside the 200 permanently sick and the 60 low weight births, we create a more comprehensive indicator of health based on a larger number of cases. By the same token, in addition, the greater is the coverage of a ward's population as a result. A final consideration is that death, chronic sickness and birthweight do not reflect an area's health in quite the same way. From a temporal point of view, mortality is an indication of past conditions, circumstances, experience and behaviour more than present or recent ones. With regard to birthweight the emphasis is the other way around; and for permanent sickness it is arguably somewhere between the two. Now this variation is a useful feature of the three indicators in themselves; but it also enhances the comprehensive nature of the Overall Health Index, for it brings together present, recent and longer-term influences on the health of an area's population. Would that the principle could be further extended in practice.

The purpose of the Overall Health Index is not, then, to supplant consideration of mortality, sickness and low birthweight individually: rather, it is to supplement and summarise these three dimensions of health, and to lead into a discussion of each in turn. In order to combine the three separate health measures into one overall index, we have employed the well-established Z-scores technique (see Appendix 2). This has been used by the Department of the Environment (1983) and by Jarman (1983, 1984). A simpler alternative technique having similar results is that of cumulative ranking (see Townsend *et al.*, 1984).

3.2 THE CONSTRUCTION OF A MEASURE OF DEPRIVATION

This study is about health inequalities, or the unequal distribution of health in one region. However, health does not exist in a social vacuum, for it is the manual working class, and within that class the poorer and more deprived sections of the population, those with fewest resources at their disposal, who generally experience the worst health (the Black Report, 1980). To provide a socio-economic framework within which to set our data on health, therefore, we have selected certain indicators derived from the 1981 Census which allow us to provide an operational definition of deprivation. Much of what we have said about the difficulty of encapsulating health through statistical indicators applies equally to 'deprivation', a concept which takes a variety of forms and has different meanings (Townsend, 1979; Brown and Madge 1982). Some recent attempts to create an operational definition of deprivation have rested on confusing foundations and have led to confusing results (notably, Department of the Environment, 1983). Before we put into operation our own definition of deprivation, it is therefore all the more important that we clarify both the meanings of deprivation and the scope of indicators which are used to measure or reflect it.

In contrast with the limited number of available health indicators, there is at first sight no shortage of indicators of deprivation. The problem here is of a different kind — namely, the selection of a coherent set of indicators, or those which reflect a clear and preferably specific meaning of deprivation. The compilation of different measures of deprivation has been pursued energetically in recent years (e.g. Holterman, 1975; Department of the Environment, 1983; Jarman, 1983, 1984, 1985; Scott-Samuel, 1983, 1984; GLC, 1985; Thunhurst, 1985a, b). Yet too often there may have been a tendency to 'trawl' for possible measures without enough regard being paid to the overall sociological rationale for the selection. All recent examples pose problems and we will illustrate some of the problems from both official and independent measures. Two indices of deprivation have been put forward, for example, by the Department of the Environment and by Professor Jarman. Both studies combine indicators of conditions and people in a composite index. The Department of the Environment produces the finding that the ten most deprived local authorities in England are all in London, with none from the Northern Region in the worst 20[2] (1983). In addition, Professor Jarman finds that seven of the ten most deprived health districts in England are in London, with none in the Northern

Region (Jarman, 1985). However, Jarman uses the term 'under-privileged' rather than 'deprived' and carefully points out that his index is primarily 'an attempt to measure general practitioners' assessments of their workload or pressure on their services' (private communication; see also Jarman, 1984, p. 1592). Nonetheless, there are eight components of the index, which is the same number as in the Department of Environment index and six of these eight are also identical or nearly the same. The pattern of results produced by the two measures is not dissimilar.

What stands out from these measures is that the 'most deprived areas in England' do not include districts drawn from the Northern Region and this flies in the face of most observation and experience. In resolving this paradox, clearly a major issue is how deprivation has to be conceived, and how best that conception can be related to such official statistics as are available. Results such as those produced in the two studies mentioned here are only achieved by selecting certain indicators the relation of some of which to depriva-tion is either indirect or contentious.

The approach adopted in this study may be summarised as follows. Indicators of deprivation are sometimes direct and sometimes indirect, sometimes representing conditions or states and sometimes representing the victims of those conditions or states. From a sociological perspective it is important to distinguish between the measurement of deprivation in different areas and the kind of people experiencing that deprivation. Otherwise there is a danger of treating social categories like age, ethnicity and single parenthood as causes of the phenomenon under study. It is, we believe, mistaken to treat being black, old and alone, or a single parent, as part of the definition of deprivation. Even if many among these minorities are deprived, some are not, and the point is to find out how many *are* deprived rather than operate as if all were in that condition. It is the form which their deprivation takes and not their status which has to be measured. Yet it is precisely the indicators that merely reflect minorities at risk of deprivation to which the Department of the Environment and other studies give considerable weight. Three of the six measures combined in the Department of the Environment index (1983), and five of the eight combined in Jarman's index (1984, 1985) are of this kind. Moreover, this particular choice of indicators can be shown to determine the outcome; variables such as single parenthood, population loss and, above all, ethnicity each tend to produce high scores for a number of the inner London Boroughs, and relatively low scores for

35

Northern districts. This will be clarified below. More generally, the selection and combination of deprivation indicators has major implications for the ranking of areas. Hitherto, these implications do not appear to have been given sufficient weight.

Our approach is also built upon the conceptual distinction between material and social forms of deprivation. Material deprivation entails the lack of the goods, services, resources, amenities and physical environment which are customary, or at least widely approved in the society under consideration. Social deprivation, on the other hand, is non-participation in the roles, relationships, customs, functions, rights and responsibilities implied by membership of a society and its sub-groups. People are socially isolated, withdrawn or excluded, for whatever reason. Such deprivation may be attributed to the effects of racism, sexism and ageism and other features of the social structures of modern economies, for example, and not only to what are taken to be the more 'natural' outcomes of ageing, or individual life processes like disablement and family bereavement. Both 'material' and 'social' deprivation can also be divided into different forms or sub-elements (see Townsend, 1987). In this study we concentrate on measures of material deprivation.

Four indicators from the 1981 Census have been selected to represent material deprivation. These have been combined in an Overall Deprivation Index, on the same lines as our Overall Health Index, with equal weights given to each measure. The four chosen variables are:

(1) *Unemployment.* The percentage of economically active residents aged 16–59/64 who are unemployed.
(2) *Car ownership.* The percentage of private households who do not possess a car.
(3) *Home ownership.* The percentage of private households not owner occupied.
(4) *Overcrowding.* The percentage of private households with more than one person per room.

Unemployment, at least at the present time, is to the assessment of material deprivation what mortality rates are to the measurement of health: an indicator which is acknowledged to be very wide in scope as well as reliable — for it reflects a great deal more than the lack of access to earned income and the facilities of employment, in that it carries implications for a general lack of material resources and the insecurity to which this gives rise. In short, unemployment is a harbinger of other misfortune.

The lack of a car is perhaps a more controversial choice, for it is not a clearcut and direct reflection of household or individual deprivation as such. However, a number of studies show that it is probably the best surrogate for current income. Not only does a family have to buy or replace a car to own one, but it also has to pay for licence, insurance and MOT, together with maintenance and repair. All this represents a substantial proportion of income. The indicator also pinpoints generally low income areas (in the absence of direct indicators of such data as children receiving free school meals and electricity disconnections, both of which were used in the Bristol study by Townsend *et al.*, 1984).

Non-owner occupation reflects lack of wealth as well as income, and therefore the scope for choice in the crucial sector of the housing market. It is perhaps a more appropriate surrogate for income in a longer-term sense than car possession provides. Taken together these two criteria offer a fairly good reflection of income levels in different areas.

Finally, overcrowding gives a more general guide to living circumstances and housing conditions. An alternative indicator often used would be the proportion of households without exclusive use of basic amenities such as bath and indoor toilet. But this has been demonstrated to be no longer widely representative of poor housing. Many council estates with such basic amenities in every household have nonetheless often been shown to hold large numbers of flats or houses in poor structural condition or with poor facilities otherwise; accordingly its usefulness as one of the main indicators seemed to be small. As a priority indicator of poor housing the more broadly based yardstick of overcrowding seemed preferable. This overcrowding indicator also helps to balance that on housing tenure, bearing in mind that in the present day owner occupation by no means always represents substantial command of resources and may be partly determined by somewhat varying traditions of provision of public housing. Altogether, the index we have put together is not extensive, nor is it ideal, but we believe it is a clear and coherent index which makes good use of census variables.

As with the health indicators, the overall picture of deprivation will be presented first, going on to look briefly at each indicator separately. Other census measures of deprivation are not completely excluded from the analysis, and will be brought into the later presentation of evidence. However, the main emphasis will be on the four chosen criteria. One point deserves to be stressed: not all deprived people live in deprived wards, just as not everybody in a ward ranked as deprived themselves count as deprived.

Missing from this discussion to date has been any reference to social class — or more accurately, occupational class. The proportion of households with a head who is semi-skilled or unskilled (Classes IV and V), or the latter alone, is often included as an indicator of deprivation in census-based studies of area inequalities (Jarman, 1983, 1984, 1985; Thunhurst, 1985b). There is of course an important sense in which occupational class and deprivation are closely related and can almost be treated as different elements of the same phenomenon; and it is not hard to see why the proportion of 'unskilled is taken as a guide to deprivation. However, the same objection can be made to the inclusion of 'low' class as a measure of deprivation as to the inclusion of ethnicity, single parenthood or pensioner status. These are categories within the population which are especially prone to forms of deprivation, but should not be incorporated in the definition of deprivation as such. Moreover, if these categories of people are included in the definition, we are denied the opportunity of discovering how many of them are deprived in various ways. This is most feasible in the case of occupational class, where it is more important to see precisely how deprivation is distributed in relation to class than to treat one as an aspect of the other. Consequently, in this study data on occupational class will be handled separately from those on deprivation. This will allow different facets of the interrelationship between health, deprivation and class to be explored.

3.3 THE WARD AS A UNIT OF ANALYSIS

Despite the value of Health District or local authority level statistics, these administrative areas are still too large to facilitate scientific exposition and analysis: wide internal variations are concealed. Inevitably, quite large sub-areas will have very different characteristics, and will counterbalance each other in producing overall or average figures for the area as a whole which can be misleading. Thus, district health authorities in the North range from 87,000 to 300,000 in population; while local authorities, which in some cases are much more homogeneous, still range from just under 25,000 up to 299,000. It is helpful, therefore, to focus on smaller areas, and although in theory there are numerous possibilities, in practice little choice is afforded.

This study takes the local authority ward, of which there were

678 in the region at the start of 1984, as the basic unit of analysis. The advantages of selecting this unit are chiefly practical and policy-related. Wards are relevant areas to local authorities and to district health authorities. Information produced about wards feeds in readily to local political and planning processes. There is also one other primary consideration. In England (but not in Scotland) the ward is the smallest area for which it is realistically possible to match 1981 Census data and the postcoded health data on births and deaths (the two foundations of this study), given that the 1981 Census geography was not postcode-based (see Appendix 1).

However, there is a price to pay for taking the ward as a unit of study. It may be a relevant area for administrators, planners and politicians, but it suffers from the disadvantage that its boundaries may have been drawn arbitrarily, in order to arrive at an appropriate number of voters rather than to identify a 'natural' community. This means that the ward population is often far from homogeneous. Thus, even an analysis as localised as one at ward level should not be expected to produce an ideal or complete picture of the extent of privilege or deprivation. A particular ward may represent the administrative amalgamation of socially dissimilar localities, or conversely, a single community may be split between two or even three wards. A further drawback is that ward boundaries are redrawn at frequent intervals, depending on changes in the voting population. This can frustrate analysis of trends because administrative definitions of an area, and the size and composition of its population, may be different after a short span of years.

One other disadvantage of using the ward as the basic geographical unit is the variability in the size of its population. The smallest ward among the 678 has a population of 500, the largest 15,500. However, only 6 per cent of wards have populations below 1,000, and one-quarter below 2,000. To counteract the problem of size in the smallest wards, the data on births and deaths cover three successive years, in order to give as sound a base as possible for analysis, and to help reduce the danger that evidence for a single year can be quite unrepresentative for a number of wards. When presenting data for individual wards, we will generally cite the actual number of health-related events on which the quoted rates are based. Furthermore, in Chapter 4 we present evidence for clusters of adjacent wards in certain areas. Clustering wards in this way offers a valuable check on the significance of high or low rates in particular wards, and makes it possible to have greater confidence in concluding that an area has an extreme health experience.

It would be wrong, however, to regard the ward as an inappropriate and unsatisfactory unit. In the first place, wards frequently do correspond quite well with socially homogeneous or locally meaningful boundaries in both urban and rural areas, though perhaps more often in the latter. Secondly, there is commonly no consensus in any case as to the boundaries of a community. Opinion tends to vary, and people are always more certain of the core of a place than of its edges. Thirdly, as will become apparent, wards do adequately serve the purpose of this study in highlighting the extent of inequality in health, even if there are areas which would probably have featured very differently in the conclusions had the boundaries themselves been drawn differently. Finally, there are at present no feasible alternatives (at least for measures of health and deprivation during inter-censal periods) and, even if there were, in technical terms it seems unlikely that they would have the immediate relevance of wards. (It is of course possible to group wards on the basis of social characteristics — see, for example, Webber, 1977 and Fox *et al.*, 1984.)

This study is based on the ward boundaries current at the start of 1984. Since the 1981 Census ward boundaries have been redrawn in several authorities (Tyne and Wear, Carlisle DC, Sedgefield DC, Teesdale DC and Wear Valley DC). For this reason the Census data were reassembled for the 198 of the 678 wards which have been constituted since the 1981 Census.

Part Two:

Description

4

The Distribution of Poor Health in the Northern Region

This chapter presents evidence on poor health in the 678 wards in the Northern Region, starting with the overall pattern, as produced by the health index, which was described in the previous chapter. Poor health is spread unevenly. Table 4.1 lists the twelve wards with the worst and best overall health (excluding wards with relatively small populations) giving separate details of their premature mortality, permanent sickness and low birthweight, and showing how high each ranks in terms of overall deprivation. Three of the wards with poorest health are in Easington and another four on Teesside. The full list from which Table 4.1 is drawn is set out in Appendix 6. It illustrates the value of creating an overall measure of health. Thus, for example, the larger wards of Tyne and Wear produce numerous cases on all three health criteria (making a total of nearly 600 health events or experiences, for example, in West City); but in small wards, it is the combination of the three criteria and the enlargement of the number of cases which that represents, which strengthens confidence in the validity of the overall ranking.

In wards with the worst health overall, there is also evidence of poor health in each individual respect, according to all three criteria. With only one exception the twelve wards with poorest health feature in the region's worst 20 per cent of wards on all three counts. By eye the reader can see that on criteria of health the two sets of wards are quite distinct. In only one instance do any of the wards with poor health compare favourably with any of the wards with good health. Willington East has a lower female SMR than Beckermet and Glebe. Against that paradoxical comparison there are many others where mortality, permanent sickness and low birthweight are twice or even three or four times as high as in the wards with relatively good health.

Table 4.1: The twelve wards with the worst and best Overall Health in the Northern Region with populations over 3,000

Rank	Ward name	District	Population	Deaths, 0–64 persons 1981–3		Deaths, 0–64 1981–3 Male	Female	Permanently sick or disabled persons 1981		Low birth-weight babies (under 2800g.) 1982–4		Overall deprivation rank
				SMR	No.	SMR	SMR	%	No.	%	No.	
WORST HEALTH												
1	Wheatley Hill	Easington	3754	159	52	147	175	4.9	145	24.0	23	124
2	West City	Newcastle	9267	191	136	201	159	5.1	369	18.6	91	3
4	Bede	Gateshead	9235	197	147	206	177	4.4	314	19.9	87	25
5	Woodhouse Close	Wear Valley	5505	167	81	138	214	5.4	227	19.8	49	13
7	Portrack & Tilery	Stockton	6042	200	100	187	218	5.3	256	15.3	45	48
8	Willington East	Wear Valley	3566	127	42	143	98	5.1	150	23.7	28	141
9	Deneside	Easington	4860	139	59	147	123	5.4	204	20.2	35	28
10	Shotton	Easington	4256	141	52	117	179	7.0	235	13.4	18	87
11	St Hilda's	Middlesbrough	3844	180	57	178	170	4.4	128	18.4	46	10
12	South Bank	Langbaurgh	6308	193	88	189	191	3.6	156	19.3	102	21
13	Sandwith	Copeland	3198	211	53	193	236	3.6	86	16.8	27	40
14	Owton	Hartlepool	6296	182	91	179	188	4.1	189	18.3	62	4
BEST HEALTH												
622	Beckermet	Copeland	3057	83	21	62	117	0.9	21	9.6	10	489
626	Glebe	Stockton	5914	83	31	72	100	1.0	41	8.9	20	655
637	Park West	Darlington	3295	72	20	96	37	1.1	30	9.2	7	627
640	Morpeth North	Castle Morpeth	3329	95	22	97	93	0.5	11	8.3	8	659
642	Marton	Middlesbrough	5086	91	29	90	92	0.6	23	8.5	19	641
643	St Mary's	North Tyneside	8937	69	49	70	65	1.0	65	9.8	21	669
644	Grange	South Lakeland	3079	83	22	85	88	1.4	37	6.1	4	639
646	Belmont	Durham	3892	73	17	81	58	0.6	15	10.1	15	670
650	Parkside	Blyth Valley	7106	64	19	49	91	0.6	27	10.8	69	584
662	Neville's Cross	Durham	4105	49	16	39	66	1.3	43	7.6	10	654
667	Hummersknott	Darlington	3666	44	15	58	23	1.2	35	7.5	5	672
668	Hutton	Langbaurgh	4014	41	11	40	41	0.6	18	7.1	9	676

4.1 OVERALL POOR HEALTH

Table 4.1 illustrates how poor health can be documented at ward level, and identifies the particular wards which, according to our chosen criteria, experience the worst health of all. A more representative method of displaying the evidence on the unequal distribution of ill-health in the Region is to be found in Figure 4.1. This is based on an analysis of the 136 wards at either end of the health spectrum, which comprise the Region's worst and best 20 per cent of wards. In it the proportion of a local authority's population living in wards ranked among the worst and best quintile in the Region is shown. The benefit of this form of presentation, which is used for all the health and deprivation variables, is that it highlights the extent of local concentrations of poor health or good health, yet within the more familiar context of the local government district. An advantage over simple district-level information is, of course, that by this method the averaging effect of gross data is minimised, as a district picture is built up from its component small areas. At the risk of labouring the point, however, it should be recalled that not everyone in a ward with a bad health record will themselves experience poor health, any more than everyone will be healthy in a ward with a good health record.

As Figure 4.1 shows, Easington has the greatest proportion of its population living in wards defined as experiencing bad health — over 50 per cent. It is also a district without any ward among the best quintile in the Region, giving a transparently clear demonstration of just how severe Easington's health problems are. This is a theme to which we shall return often in this chapter. Hartlepool, Middlesbrough and Wear Valley follow Easington, with between 45 and 48 per cent of their residents living in wards with bad health records. Gateshead and Newcastle come next, with just over 40 per cent in this category. All these districts stand out as possessing large and serious concentrations of ill-health.

In one sense, however, Easington and Middlesbrough stand apart. If attention is focused upon the worst 10 per cent of wards in the Region, rather than the worst 20 per cent, these two districts emerge with even more pronounced concentrations of ill-health — for in both places, around 40 per cent of the population are to be found in wards ranked within this extreme category: 42 per cent in Middlesbrough and 39 per cent in Easington. No other district comes close to such proportions. A particularly strong contrast may be noted here between Middlesbrough on the one hand, and

Figure 4.1: Overall health. Proportion of each district's population living in wards ranked among the best and worst fifth in the Northern Region

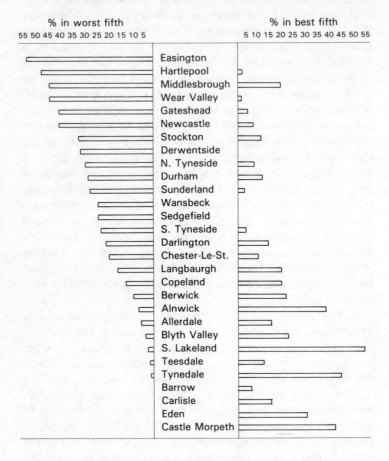

Note: Districts are ranked on the basis of the proportion of population in the worst fifth of wards.

Sunderland and South Tyneside on the other. Whereas no less than ten of the 25 wards in Middlesbrough are to be found among the worst decile in the region, only one of the 45 wards in Sunderland and South Tyneside has a health record bad enough to place it in this group. The severity of ill-health in large pockets of Middlesbrough, and the relatively moderate level of ill-health generally in the worst wards in Sunderland and South Tyneside, constitute a contrast to which we shall frequently return in this study.

At the other end of the health spectrum, South Lakeland stands out as having a very high proportion of the 'healthiest' wards, with Tynedale, Castle Morpeth and Alnwick not far behind. It is also worth noting two contrasting patterns. In certain districts, sizeable proportions of the population live in wards at the two poles of the health spectrum. Middlesbrough is an excellent example of this pattern, for alongside its large number of wards with a bad health record, there are also several with a good enough record to rank within the Region's best quintile. In differing degrees this pattern is discernible in Darlington, Langbaurgh, Copeland and Berwick. However, there are several districts where the overwhelming majority of people live in wards which rank in the middle ranges of the distribution. In Carlisle and Barrow there are no wards with health poor enough to place them among the Region's worst; yet conversely neither district has more than a very few wards at the opposite end of the spectrum.

4.2 MORTALITY

Data about deaths, derived from death returns, offer scope for detailed analyses of differences between populations. The generally high mortality in the Northern Region is reflected in the fact that 416 of the 678 wards (representing 61 per cent of wards but 70 per cent of total population) fare worse than the England and Wales average for deaths under the age of 65 years (i.e. SMRs over 100).

Figure 4.2 shows the regional distribution of the wards at the two extremes of mortality, ranked by local authority. This figure makes abundantly clear the extent to which Middlesbrough and Hartlepool more than anywhere else suffer from high levels of premature mortality. In both these cases, one half of the population lives in wards which are among the worst fifth in the Region. Darlington and Easington follow, though it is important to note that Darlington's wards with relatively high mortality fall largely in the lower reaches

Figure 4.2: Premature mortality. Proportion of each district's population living in wards ranked among the best and worst fifth in the Northern Region

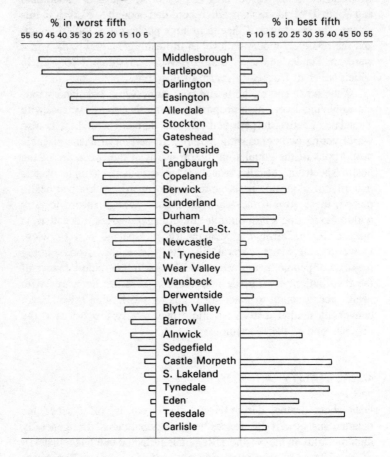

Note: Districts are ranked on the basis of the proportion of population in the worst fifth of wards.

of the Region's worst quintile, whereas many of Easington's are close to the extreme. Outside the most heavily populated parts of the north-east, Allerdale, Copeland, and, perhaps surprisingly, Berwick, all emerge as having significant pockets of premature mortality. At the oppposite end of mortality experience, South Lakeland has more than half of its population living in wards which are among the best quintile in the Region. No other district matches that, although Teesdale, Castle Morpeth, Tynedale, Alnwick and Eden make up a group of six largely rural districts where premature mortality levels are generally low.

An important contrast is also evident in Figure 4.2 between the districts of Cleveland on the one hand, and Tyne and Wear on the other. Three of Cleveland's four districts outrank the worst of the Tyne and Wear districts (Gateshead), so far as the proportion of people living in the worst quintile band is concerned; and this is just one indication that high mortality is more widely spread in Cleveland than Tyne and Wear. To give another striking example of this: one ward in five in Cleveland has a rate of premature mortality that is 50 per cent or more above the national average (SMRs of 150 and above); in Tyne and Wear that ratio is just 1 in 14.

Table 4.2: Premature mortality in Tyne and Wear and Cleveland: based on ward groupings by district, 1981–3 deaths

| District | SMRs | | | |
	Worst quarter	Second worst quarter	Second best quarter	Best quarter
Middlesbrough	170	146	115	86
Langbaurgh	167	127	104	82
Hartlepool	165	139	117	87
Gateshead	160	128	115	99
Stockton	155	123	101	86
Newcastle	155	122	108	93
North Tyneside	144	117	104	81
South Tyneside	138	124	113	101
Sunderland	136	123	113	96

Notes: Districts are ranked on the basis of the SMR for the worst quarter of their wards. For the SMRs, England and Wales = 100.

This comparison between Cleveland and Tyne and Wear is taken further in Table 4.2. In this case the wards in each district have been divided into four bands on the basis of their premature mortality, and an SMR calculated for each quarter bloc. Consequently, the full distribution is illustrated here. The degree to which Cleveland bears the brunt of the highest mortality is confirmed by the very high figures in the worst band of wards. This method of presentation depicts clearly, for instance, the scale of the mortality problem in the worst wards in Langbaurgh; but it also shows that mortality in the second worst band of wards in Middlesbrough and Hartlepool is actually higher than in the worst band of some Tyne and Wear districts. Within the former metropolitan county, Gateshead and Newcastle experience by some distance the highest premature mortality, with levels comparable with Cleveland. However, the worst band in the other three districts reveals significantly lower levels, especially in South Tyneside and Sunderland. These two just do not experience the very high rates of premature death observable in all four Cleveland districts and also in Gateshead and Newcastle. At the same time, South Tyneside and Sunderland manifestly do not experience low mortality levels. South Tyneside, indeed, is the one district under consideration here with the SMR for the best band of wards above 100. Sunderland's is not much lower. In both districts the mortality gradient from the worst wards to the best is relatively slight, and even the second best band of wards experience raised mortality levels. In contrast, in Cleveland, a much more pronounced mortality gradient is apparent, with steep declines from one band to the next. Moreover, mortality in the best band is lower in Cleveland than anywhere in Tyne and Wear with the exception of North Tyneside, illuminating the extent to which this county combines extremes.

Perhaps the sharpest illustration of high premature mortality in Cleveland is the continuous band of wards along the south side of the Tees, shown in Figure 4.3a. Extending from Thornaby (Victoria Ward) right across Middlesbrough and South Bank to the mouth of the Tees (Coatham Ward), this bloc of 15 adjoining wards contains a population of 86,000. Not one of the wards in this bloc has an individual SMR of less than 140 for deaths under 65; and the combined SMR is 164. This represents a total of 370 deaths per year of people under 65, of which 145 may be regarded as 'excess deaths' — in other words, deaths which would not have occurred had this area experienced the mortality of England and Wales as a whole. Only one other area in the Northern Region covering a population of comparable scale has such an extremely high level of premature mortality. Indeed, there cannot be more than a very few such areas in the country as a whole. Straddling the Tyne, a bloc of six wards in the centres of Newcastle and Gateshead (Moorside and West City

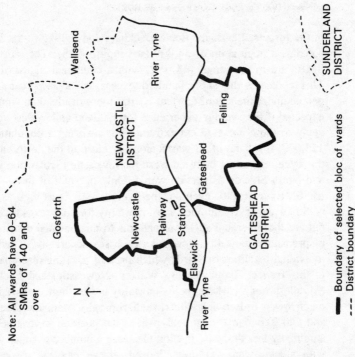

Figure 4.3a: Bloc of 15 wards in Cleveland (south bank of River Tees) with very high premature mortality

Note: All wards have 0–64 SMRs of 140 and over

— Boundary of selected bloc of wards
— · — County boundary
- - - District boundary

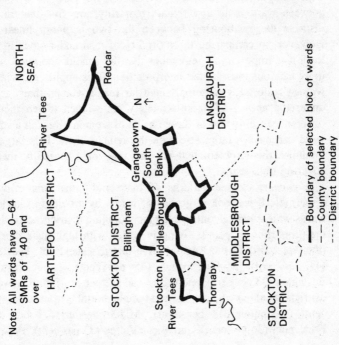

Figure 4.3b: Bloc of six wards in Newcastle and Gateshead with very high premature mortality

Note: All wards have 0–64 SMRs of 140 and over

— Boundary of selected bloc of wards
- - - District boundary

in the former; Bensham, Bede, Deckham and Felling in the latter) contains a population of 54,000 (see Figure 4.3b). The individual SMRs are in the range 148–197, with a combined figure of 170. This represents almost one hundred 'excess deaths' each year among people under the age of 65 (that is, 100 more deaths than would be expected if the average experience for England and Wales were to apply to these areas). Less extreme, but covering a population of 125,000, is a band of 13 wards along or close to the north bank of the Tyne, extending between western Newcastle (Scotswood ward) and North Shields (Riverside ward). Only one-half of these wards has SMRs over 140: even so, the overall SMR is as high as 142.

So far we have examined ward mortality for both sexes together, but are there perhaps different patterns to this unequal distribution of premature mortality if we take each sex separately? There are individual localities or wards which present puzzling discrepancies in this respect. Examples are Walker (Newcastle) and Beckfield (Middlesbrough), where men's mortality is very high and women's much lower; or Berwick Hills (Middlesbrough), Mandale (Stockton) and Old Trimdon (Sedgefield) where the position is reversed. In admittedly less dramatic fashion there are a number of other wards with a significant variation. Indeed, if we plot the association between ward male and female mortality, we find that in most districts the relationship between the two is not a linear one. However, in comparing the mortality of men and women at ward level it is important to remember that the smaller the numbers the more cautious must be the interpretation. This applies especially to women's mortality patterns, since far fewer women than men die under the age of 65 (approximately six women to ten men). A difference of only two or three deaths of women a year in a smaller ward can have a large effect on the female SMR. It is largely to minimise this problem that we use one main mortality measure covering both sexes.

However, clearer patterns of male and female mortality are discernible if we look at groups of wards by district or clusters of wards which form a continuous bloc. Ranking districts according to the proportion of people living in wards with high male mortality (the worst fifth in the Region), five districts stand out: Hartlepool (47 per cent), Middlesbrough (45 per cent), Langbaurgh and Easington (33 per cent), and Gateshead (32 per cent). Similarly, five districts stand out when we turn to female mortality: Berwick (40 per cent), Easington (38 per cent), Middlesbrough (37 per cent), Hartlepool (34 per cent), and Wear Valley (33 per cent). From this

Figure 4.4: Bloc of 22 wards in East Durham (chiefly Easington district) with high female premature mortality

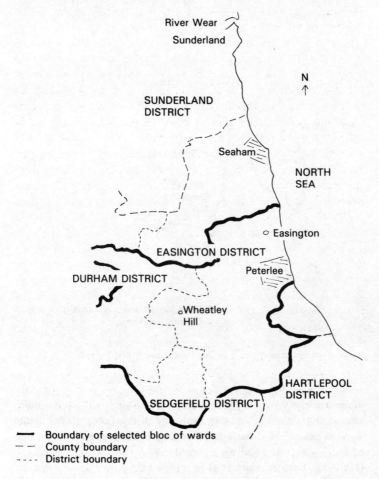

Boundary of selected bloc of wards
County boundary
District boundary

Note: Twelve wards out of 22 have female 0–64 SMRs of 140 and above; another 6 wards have SMRs between 130 and 140.

perspective, parallels between male and female mortality are more evident than major discrepancies, with the notable exception of Berwick.

We shall now examine a number of relevant blocs of adjoining wards where mortality is high, in order to compare the experience

Figure 4.5: Bloc of seven wards in West Cumbria with high premature mortality

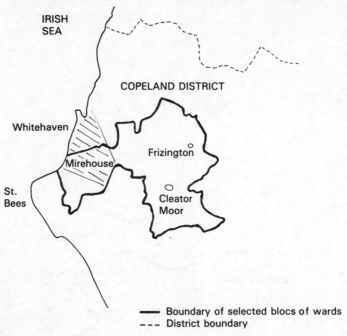

———— Boundary of selected blocs of wards
- - - District boundary

Note: 4 wards among the 7 in Copeland have SMRs over 140.

of men and women in these areas. In addition to the three blocs already mentioned (along the south side of the Tees, straddling the Tyne in central Newcastle and Gateshead, and along the north side of the Tyne), we shall also consider two further ward clusters.[3] One is in Durham, and has been selected primarily to illustrate the high female mortality in large parts of Easington and a few adjacent areas of Durham and Sedgefield. A bloc of 22 wards, covering almost all the southern half of Easington (15 of its 26 wards), four Durham and three Sedgefield wards, contains a population of 81,000 (see Figure 4.4). Its SMR for women under 65, based on 361 deaths, is 152; and all except one of the individual ward SMRs for women are over 125. In many of these wards men's mortality is also high, but the pattern is by no means as consistent as it is for women.

The other locality is in West Cumbria. The presentation of the evidence so far has concentrated on Tyneside, Teesside and much of Durham, for these are the areas where high mortality is most concentrated. However, the coastal belt in West Cumbria, split between the districts of Allerdale and Copeland, also contains significant pockets of high mortality, in and around Workington, Cleator Moor and, above all, Maryport and Whitehaven. The Aller-dale coastal belt indeed contains the one significantly large pocket of raised stillbirth and infant mortality in the Region. Moreover, Sandwith ward, on the south side of Whitehaven, has the highest mortality rate for deaths under the age of 65 in the entire Region (see Table 4.1). The bloc of wards highlighted here incorporates the southern half of Whitehaven, as well as Cleator Moor and Friz-ington, and has a population of 23,000 living in seven wards (see Figure 4.5). In this area, male and female premature mortality are both comparatively high. These examples of areas with high premature mortality are by no means exhaustive; but they do cover a representative number of the larger and more significant clusters. The evidence from these five blocs of wards is summarised in Table 4.3, which, in addition to the data on all deaths under 65, also iden-tifies mortality by selected causes. Those selected are the main causes of death: cancers (neoplasms), circulatory diseases, respiratory diseases, together with accidents, poisoning and violence, together account for approximately 85–90 per cent of all deaths under 65 years.

The very high values of the mortality ratios for almost all the causes listed in the two worst clusters (labelled South Tees and Central Tyne) tend not to be replicated in the other clusters, where the patterns are more variable. Women's mortality, however, in the Easington-Durham-Sedgefield bloc, is high for most of the specified causes. This is also the one example cited of moderately raised breast cancer levels.

Finally, two other examples of smaller clusters of wards with higher rates of premature death are also worth noting. These are from the one county which has so far not featured much in the presentation of mortality patterns — Northumberland. Northumber-land has a smaller proportion of its wards among the Region's worst 20 per cent on the criterion of premature mortality than any other county (although Cumbria has only marginally more). Nevertheless, two Northumberland towns stand out in this respect: Berwick and Ashington. Combining the five wards which make up the town of Berwick (population 11,800) produces the high SMR for all deaths under the age of 65 of 151. However, it is female mortality which is especially high (SMR 177), while male mortality is not raised to

Table 4.3: Premature mortality (0–64) in five areas of the Northern Region, 1981–3: SMRs by selected causes

Area	Sex	All deaths	140–239	162	150–9	174	390–459	460–519	E800–999
						ICD Nos.			
South Tees	M	159 (695)	176 (205)	220 (95)	150 (49)	—	160 (298)	162 (49)	129 (61)
	F	169 (416)	155 (155)	300 (45)	153 (28)	102 (28)	220 (147)	207 (37)	135 (24)
Central Tyne	M	176 (473)	170 (123)	229 (61)	144 (29)	—	168 (195)	222 (41)	196 (57)
	F	158 (245)	123 (78)	168 (16)	156 (19)	87 (15)	209 (91)	264 (29)	109 (12)
North Tyne	M	144 (936)	175 (310)	213 (142)	161 (80)	—	130 (372)	141 (64)	120 (78)
	F	138 (524)	139 (219)	273 (66)	154 (47)	84 (36)	150 (164)	168 (46)	103 (27)
Easington etc	M	125 (507)	112 (123)	109 (44)	133 (41)	—	136 (241)	168 (46)	104 (45)
	F	152 (361)	144 (143)	196 (27)	134 (25)	127 (35)	174 (114)	206 (35)	65 (11)
Whitehaven & Cleator Moor	M	145 (173)	152 (49)	168 (20)	154 (14)	—	147 (76)	122 (10)	195 (25)
	F	145 (101)	117 (34)	114 (5)	89 (5)	86 (7)	228 (44)	59 (3)	113 (6)

Notes: Actual numbers of deaths in parentheses. SMRs: England and Wales = 100.
ICD code: 140–239 — All Neoplasms; 162 — Neoplasm: trachea, bronchus and lung;
150–159 — Neoplasm: digestive system; 174 — Neoplasm: breast;
390–459 — Circulatory system diseases;
460–519 — Respiratory system diseases;
E800–999 — Accidents, poisoning and violence.

Numbers of wards per area: South Tees (15); Central Tyne (6); North Tyne (13); Easington etc. (22); Whitehaven (part) and Cleator Moor (7).

Table 4.4: Trends in mortality in England and Wales

	SMR Persons 0–64 England and Wales
1981–3	100
1950–2	149
1936–8	228
1930–2	258

anything like the same extent (SMR 136). These figures are almost exactly repeated in three adjoining Ashington wards (Central, Hirst and Park, population 11,900), where the combined SMR for both sexes is 151, and the female death rate much worse than the male (SMRs of 175 and 136 respectively). These patterns of premature mortality cannot be further analysed by the cause of death, as the total number of deaths is not sufficient to facilitate a breakdown into different categories.

One method of illustrating the significance of the higher SMRs in some parts of the North is by expressing the gap between these localities and the country as a whole in terms of the historical contrast between mortality in England and Wales at the present time and at earlier periods during this century. In Table 4.4, SMRs for England and Wales have been calculated for four periods, taking 1981–3 as the baseline. In the period from 1950 to 1952, for example, national mortality of people under the age of 65 was 50 per cent higher than it is at present (SMR 149). There are 60 wards in the region (nearly 10 per cent of the total) with SMRs for deaths under 65 at least as high as this figure; and the SMR for the 20 per cent of wards with the highest mortality now (see Appendix 5) is the same as for England and Wales in 1950–52. The upheaval of the Second World War makes it necessary to go back to the 1930s for further comparisons. The national SMR of 228 for the years 1936–8 is somewhat higher than the figures for the wards with the highest mortality in the Region today (the three highest are 211, 200 and 197). Nevertheless, the difference in relatively small.

The gap between the wards with highest and lowest premature mortality may also be portrayed in terms of national historical comparisons. With 23 wards (almost entirely rural) having SMRs below 50, and three wards having SMRs close to or above 200, premature mortality is approximately four times higher in the very worst wards of all than in the very best. Contrasting the 10 per cent

57

of wards with the highest mortality and the 10 per cent with the lowest reduces this ratio to 2.8:1 (see Chapter 6, Table 6.5). Since the level of mortality nationally for all deaths under 65 was 2.6 times higher in 1930–32 than in 1981–3, it appears that the gap between the two extreme 10 per cent bands of wards in the North is equivalent to a difference of 50 years or more in the national improvement in mortality. However, this statement requires qualification. With the decline in mortality during the twentieth century, the proportion of deaths taking place at different ages has changed. There has been a dramatic fall in the numbers dying in infancy and childhood, but a much smaller decline in death rates at later ages.

Of course areas in which there remains high mortality have shared in the reduction in infant and childhood deaths, even if not to the same extent as other parts of the country. To bring out the way in which health in. certain areas lags behind improvements in the country as a whole, we will examine how far their death rates at certain ages today correspond with rates which were common nationally many years ago. This method of presenting area mortality rates also helps to identify the number of 'avoidable' deaths — though in a social, rather than medical sense (the method was illustrated above in Figure 2.1 in Chapter 2). In Figure 4.6 the distribution by age of all deaths under 75 is compared for:

(1) England and Wales at three different periods over the last 50 years (1936–8, 1950–52 and 1981–3);
(2) two groups of two wards within one district, North Tyneside, where death rates differ very widely.

The format adopted in this figure makes it possible to show both the relative proportions of deaths in each of four age bands under 75 (0–14, 15–44, 45–64 and 65–74), and also the absolute levels of mortality, in order to emphasise the scale of historical changes and to place in context the inequalities of the present day. In North Tyneside, the adjacent wards of Riverside and Howdon have the highest mortality in the district, and both are among the Region's worst 10 per cent of wards. St Mary's and Monkseaton are likewise adjoining wards but are at the opposite pole in both district and regional terms.

In Figure 4.6, England and Wales mortality between 1981 and 1983 is taken as the standard, and for every 100 deaths under the age of 75 the breakdown by age band is illustrated. Selecting wards, as illustrated for North Tyneside, makes apparent the inequality at

Figure 4.6: The distribution by age of all deaths under 75 years in selected areas and for selected periods

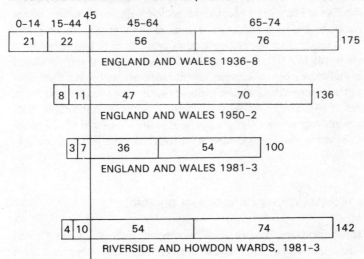

Notes: England and Wales 1981–3 = 100. All other examples have been expressed in relation to England and Wales 1981–3 experience, using direct standardisation method.

all ages, including that among those aged 0–14 and 15–44. Yet while inequalities demonstrably persist below the age of 45, it is in these earlier phases of life that historical improvements in mortality are most clearly seen. Wards like Riverside and Howdon may have about twice the mortality of St Mary's and Monkseaton through infancy and childhood; yet even so, they are very different from the national experience immediately before the Second World War.

The reverse applies over the age of 45. It is the 45–64 age range within which exists the widest current inequalities within the North and between the North and the rest of the country; and because of the large numbers of deaths involved, deaths at this age contribute most to overall differentials under the age of 75. In areas like Riverside and Howdon, 45–64 (and 65–74) mortality is identical to that of the country as a whole between 1936 and 1938. Since there are a number of large wards with worse mortality than these two, it is evident that there will be cases where mortality in the 30-year period

59

from age 45 to age 75 is comparable with the national level of the early 1930s. Moreover, the showing of adjoining localities of Tyneside like St Mary's and Monkseaton indicates the improvements which are attainable in the older as well as in the younger age ranges.

To summarise the evidence from areas of high mortality: there are wards like Riverside and Howdon, where infant and childhood mortality lags behind current national experience, but is nonetheless a great improvement on the national picture 30 years previously; in the 15–44 range, however, mortality remains comparable with national experience 30 years ago; and in the 45–64 and 65–74 range it is worse still, comparable with national experience of the late 1930s.

4.3 PERMANENT SICKNESS AND DISABILITY

The information available on permanent sickness at the Census offers less scope for analysis than either of the other two main variables; and it suffers from the potential drawback that, unlike birth and death data, it is based on self-reporting alone. Yet in the absence of other measures of morbidity covering the entire population, it is an important source of evidence. Moreover, the relatively large number of cases that this indicator is based upon, by comparison with the numbers of births or deaths, increases confidence in the reliability of patterns of variation at local level. Even more than with premature mortality, the Northern Region emerges badly: almost two-thirds (64 per cent) of the 678 wards have levels of permanent sickness worse than the England and Wales average.

The really striking feature of permanent sickness, however, is how very unequally it is distributed across the Region. Figure 4.7 brings this out clearly, showing the proportion of each district's population living in wards ranked among the extreme quintiles in the Region. It is not Cleveland which dominates the picture here, but Durham. Indeed, the seven districts which head this list were all part of County Durham as it used to be prior to the 1974 local government reorganisation. Easington heads the ranking, followed by Derwentside, Wear Valley and Durham: all four districts have over half of their population living in wards with high permanent sickness levels (i.e. in the worst quintile). Middlesbrough ranks worst among the Cleveland districts, but Gateshead, Sunderland and Newcastle all fare worse still.

At the opposite end of the scale, eleven districts in the Region are

Figure 4.7: Permanent sickness. Proportion of each district's population living in wards ranked among the best and worst fifth in the Northern Region

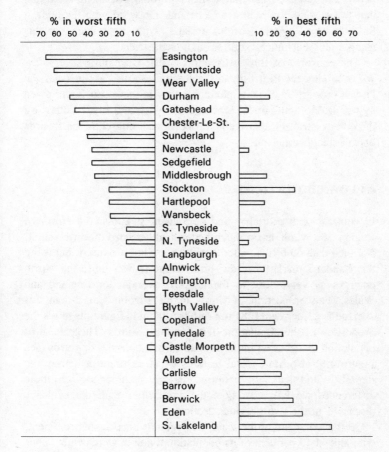

Notes: Districts are ranked on the basis of the proportion of population in the worst fifth of wards.
Range of values: in worst fifth, 3.2–7.0 per cent; in best fifth, 0.4–1.4 per cent.

either without any ward, or else have only one, in the worst quintile band. Indeed, Cumbria has only one ward in the entire county with permanent sickness sufficient to place it in the worst fifth of wards, that ward being Sandwith, in Copeland, the ward with the highest SMR in the Region. Northumberland, with eight wards in this category, is not much more strongly represented.

The converse of this distribution is that Durham has very few wards among the best fifth in the Region. South Lakeland has the largest proportion of its population living in these wards, followed by Castle Morpeth. Eden, Stockton, Berwick and Blyth Valley are the other districts with sizeable proportions living in the best wards on this health criterion.

4.4 LOW BIRTHWEIGHT

In contrast with mortality and permanent sickness, the Northern Region as a whole has a much better health record on birthweight. National data on births under 2,800 gm are not produced, but using the standard marker of low birthweight (2,500 gm), the North emerges as very close to the national average for England and Wales. The proportion of wards in the Region worse than this average is 41 per cent (281 out of 678): but this figure disguises the proportion of the population living in these wards. The pattern of population distribution in the best and worst quintiles of wards (see Figure 4.8) also has several features which distinguish it from the mortality and sickness patterns. Before commenting on these differences we will first note the similarities with the evidence discussed in the two previous sections.

At the worst end of the scale, Easington is once again prominent, with almost 40 per cent of its population living in wards with a poor record of low birthweight. This confirms the extent to which Easington consistently suffers widespread ill-health on all three indicators, and helps to account for its position at the head of the ranking in Figure 4.1 above. Cleveland districts are also once again strongly in evidence, although on this health indicator Stockton fares slightly worse than Middlesbrough, in a reversal of the mortality pattern. Wear Valley also features prominently.

Teesdale's position at the head of this list is unexpected, however. Any inference that Teesdale thus has the greatest concentration of localities with poor birthweight records should, nevertheless, be treated cautiously. On average, Teesdale's wards are the

Figure 4.8: Low birthweight. Proportion of each district's population living in wards ranked among the best and worst fifth in the Northern Region

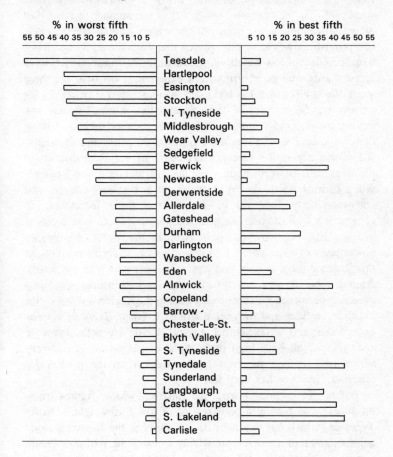

Notes: Districts are ranked on the basis of the proportion of population in the worst fifth of wards. Range of values: in worst fifth, 17.1–28.6 per cent; in best fifth, 0.0–10.8 per cent.

smallest in the Region, and the number of births below 2,800 gm in the nine wards which feature in the worst quintile are very small indeed. The total number of births below 2,800 gm from all nine wards (88) is, for example, smaller than the number in Blue Hall alone,[4] Stockton's worst ward (90 low weight births). Having made this proviso, however, it still appears that Teesdale does experience a real problem of low weight births. Most similar rural districts have a few wards with poor birthweight experience; but over the three years 1982–4 Teesdale has had more than just a few such wards, for no less than 56 per cent of its inhabitants live in wards which rank among the Region's worst. In addition, this is such a striking contrast with Teesdale's relative position on premature mortality, for on that criterion it emerges as one of the very best districts in the Region. It is worth noting that the distribution of the Region's worst fifth of wards on low birthweight is the least uneven, and correspondingly the widest, among the three indicators. In comparison with the permanent sickness distribution, where eleven districts had no ward (or only one) in the worst quintile, or premature mortality, where four districts were in such a position, in this instance there is only one case (Carlisle, with a single ward). Among other things, this broader distribution ensures somewhat greater prominence for rural wards among the Region's worst — for example, in Eden and Alnwick districts. Even so, Teesdale is quite exceptional; and while South Lakeland, Castle Morpeth, Tynedale and Alnwick all have high proportions of people living in wards which rank among the best in the Region on the birthweight criterion, Teesdale has very few.

Within Tyne and Wear, the district which figures most prominently as having a poor record of low birthweight is North Tyneside, which has seven of its 20 wards in the Region's worst quintile, and thus a much more widely spread pattern of poor health experience than it has on mortality or permanent sickness. One interesting facet of the Tyne and Wear picture is, in fact, the extent of the divergence between the five districts — for in contrast with North Tyneside, South Tyneside and Sunderland both have extremely low proportions of their populations living in wards which are among the worst in the Region in terms of low birthweight. This pattern is also brought out in Table 4.5, which compares the Tyne and Wear and Cleveland districts, looking at the percentages of births under 2,800 gm in four bands of wards, from the worst to the best, in each district. The relatively unfavourable position of Stockton, Hartlepool and North Tyneside, in relation to Langbaurgh,

Table 4.5: Low birthweight in Tyne and Wear and Cleveland, based on ward groupings by district, 1982–4 births

| District | % live births below 2,800 gm | | | |
	Worst quarter	Second worst quarter	Second best quarter	Best quarter
Stockton	20.7	17.8	15.5	12.4
North Tyneside	20.0	17.0	14.2	11.1
Middlesbrough	19.7	16.9	13.9	11.5
Gateshead	19.7	15.6	13.1	12.0
Hartlepool	19.7	17.5	15.0	12.6
Newcastle	19.1	16.5	14.3	12.2
Langbaurgh	17.8	13.9	11.4	8.8
South Tyneside	17.0	15.6	14.4	10.8
Sunderland	16.6	15.1	13.3	11.2

Note: Districts are ranked on the basis of the percentage of low birthweight babies in the worst quarter of their wards.

South Tyneside and Sunderland, comes across quite clearly.

Finally, two small clusters of wards where a significant incidence of low birthweight babies occurs can be mentioned. Derwentside is a district with a similar proportion of its population living in wards at either end of the regional spectrum. Its wards in the worst quintile are dispersed around the district, but there is a clear concentration in and to the south of Stanley. Less pronounced than Stanley on this measure, but in a locality already identified for its premature mortality, is the Sandwith-Mirehouse cluster on the south side of Whitehaven, in Copeland.

5

The Prevalence of Deprivation in the Northern Region

Having described in the last chapter the salient features of the geographical distribution of poor health in the North, a similar analysis will now be carried out for material deprivation. The twelve wards with the greatest and least overall deprivation, according to the four chosen criteria, are listed in Table 5.1, with additional information about the proportion of households whose 'head' is of Class IV and V. The most deprived wards are concentrated within Cleveland and Tyne and Wear. Even more than with health, the two sets of wards at either extreme of the continuum are, on all four criteria, clearly distinct. Materially speaking, they are very different places. The penultimate column of the table shows that strikingly high percentages of their populations are in the poorer manual classes. Average unemployment in the twelve most deprived wards in 1981 was seven times higher than in the twelve least deprived wards — 28 per cent, compared with 4 per cent.

5.1 OVERALL DEPRIVATION

Figure 5.1 shows the distribution of ward populations which were most and least deprived by district. There are some differences from the corresponding figures describing wards with best and worst health (Figure 4.1), as well as close similarities. Middlesbrough, Newcastle, Gateshead, Hartlepool, Stockton and Derwentside all possess approximately the same proportion of their population living in the most deprived wards as they have living in the least healthy wards (as defined by inclusion in the Region's worst quintile). On the other hand, Easington and Wear Valley feature somewhat less prominently in relation to overall deprivation than they do in terms

Table 5.1: The twelve wards with the most and least Overall Deprivation in the Northern Region with populations over 3,000

Rank	Ward name	District	Population	Persons unemployed 1981 %	Households with no car 1981 %	Households not owner-occupied 1981 %	Over-crowded households 1981 %	Class IV and V households 1981 %	Overall Health rank
MOST DEPRIVED									
1	Pallister	Middlesbrough	5803	30.9	76.1	92.2	13.4	54.2	41
2	Thorntree	Middlesbrough	10410	36.7	76.6	95.9	8.3	53.9	40
3	West City	Newcastle	9267	29.8	84.3	97.1	7.9	49.5	2
4	Owton	Hartlepool	6296	29.7	73.2	95.2	8.4	46.9	14
5	Walker	Newcastle	11055	23.2	81.6	93.3	8.6	41.4	89
6	Church Lane	Langbaurgh	4612	28.4	68.2	91.7	8.9	40.5	25
7	Felling	Gateshead	9928	22.1	72.3	88.0	10.8	37.1	34
8	Town End Farm	Sunderland	11686	26.7	69.2	92.7	8.6	36.2	136
9	Monkchester	Newcastle	9289	21.1	78.3	88.7	8.9	42.1	63
10	St Hilda's	Middlesbrough	3844	32.9	78.2	66.8	9.4	47.4	11
11	Hardwick	Stockton	6015	25.9	69.5	96.4	7.8	41.0	52
12	Scotswood	Newcastle	10667	26.5	73.7	68.2	12.3	38.8	24

Table 5.1 continued

Rank	Ward name	District	Population	Persons unemployed 1981 %	Households with no car 1981 %	Households not owner-occupied 1981 %	Over-crowded households 1981 %	Class IV and V households 1981 %	Overall Health rank
LEAST DEPRIVED									
659	Morpeth North	Castle Morpeth	3329	5.1	17.6	15.4	0.7	4.9	640
660	Hartburn	Stockton	7716	6.9	13.8	3.1	0.9	11.6	525
661	Cleadon and East Boldon	South Tyneside	8313	5.9	17.8	8.0	0.7	5.5	588
668	Hawcoat	Barrow	5713	3.8	17.7	2.5	0.8	8.2	559
669	St Mary's	North Tyneside	8937	5.2	18.4	6.4	0.2	2.9	643
670	Belmont	Durham	3892	3.5	9.1	5.9	1.0	8.3	646
672	Hummersknott	Darlington	3666	4.8	15.4	7.6	0.2	1.1	667
674	Mowden	Darlington	3932	4.0	20.4	7.0	0.1	6.5	524
675	Newton Hall	Durham	5699	3.1	11.2	6.2	0.5	11.6	531
676	Hutton	Langbaurgh	4014	4.6	5.7	6.4	0.2	4.7	674
677	Ponteland West	Castle Morpeth	3197	3.5	5.9	6.5	0.3	3.7	585
678	Ponteland South	Castle Morpeth	3098	1.9	4.5	2.1	0.1	0.0	601

Figure 5.1: Overall deprivation. Proportion of each district's population living in wards ranked among the best and worst fifth in the Northern Region

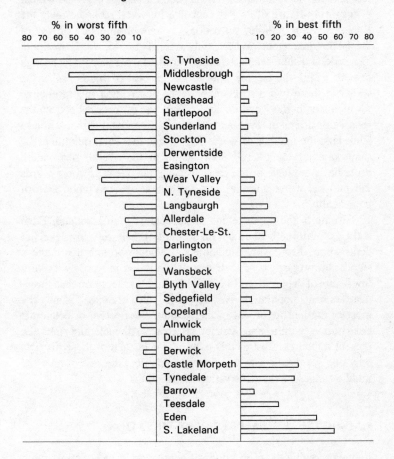

Note: Districts are ranked on the basis of the proportion of population in the worst fifth of wards.

of health; whereas conversely South Tyneside and Sunderland figure much more prominently in relation to deprivation. South Tyneside, indeed, has the vast majority of its people living in deprived wards: a staggering figure of 75 per cent live in wards ranked among the Region's worst quintile, yet it does not rate prominently on any of the health indicators. Where only one of the 45 wards in South Tyneside and Sunderland has an overall health record bad enough to rank within the Region's worst 10 per cent of wards, 14 of the wards in these two districts experience deprivation severe enough for inclusion in the worst decile. In fact, one difference between the relative positions of Tyne and Wear and Cleveland is that while in Cleveland the number of wards falling into the worst quintile is the same whether the overall poor health or the overall deprivation criterion is applied, in the case of Tyne and Wear 15 more wards fall into the worst quintile on the criterion of deprivation than of poor health.

Turning to the opposite end of the scale, South Lakeland, Eden and Castle Morpeth stand out on account of their very low levels of deprivation. Moreover, Stockton and Middlesbrough also have a significant proportion of their population living in wards with very low levels of deprivation. In Middlesbrough's case, more than three-quarters of its population lives in wards which are either among the most or the least deprived in the Region, a reflection of economic polarisation within one district. Barrow, Alnwick and Berwick present a total contrast to this pattern, for in each of these districts only one ward falls into the extreme quintiles: the rest occupy the middle ranges of the deprivation distribution.

5.2 INDIVIDUAL MEASURES OF DEPRIVATION

Figures showing the proportions of population in each district living in the most and least deprived wards in the Region are given in Appendix 5. Two districts stand out as experiencing severe deprivation on all four criteria of deprivation: Middlesbrough and, above all, South Tyneside. Hartlepool, Easington and the four remaining Tyne and Wear districts each figure prominently on at least three of the deprivation indicators.

There is a contrast between the ranking on the unemployment indicator and the other three indicators: not only because unemployment is acute in places like Derwentside, but more especially because unemployment is more acute in Cleveland districts than

Tyne and Wear. At the 1981 Census, for example, nine Middlesbrough wards were found to be experiencing an unemployment rate
of over 25 per cent, but only one South Tyneside ward reached that
figure. Indeed, however bad unemployment was in Tyne and Wear
in 1981, it was worse in Cleveland; and this pattern has continued
in the years since then. Recent figures show that Cleveland at
present experiences the highest unemployment of any county in
Britain, with Tyne and Wear third after Merseyside, and Durham
not far behind (Department of Employment, 1984, 1985). Within
Tyne and Wear, South Tyneside and Sunderland have the highest
unemployment (ibid., 1985; Tyne and Wear County Council, 1985)
— but the figures mask some real differences. In South Tyneside the
local pattern is uniform. Thus, in July 1985 no postcode sector there
had unemployment exceeding 30 per cent. In contrast, there is a
more varied local pattern in both Sunderland and Newcastle, where
more than a dozen postcode sectors in all had an unemployment rate
of over 30 per cent, with one area in each district having a rate over
40 per cent in July 1985 (Tyne and Wear County Council, 1985).
In Teesside, local unemployment rates cover a wide range, but the
worst affected inner city areas, particularly along the south side of
the river, experience levels that are still higher than in Sunderland
and west Newcastle, with 40 per cent unemployment in wards or
postcode sectors no longer uncommon.[5]

The case of Langbaurgh is instructive. Despite containing three
of the most consistently deprived — and unhealthy — wards in
Teesside (Grangetown, South Bank and Church Lane), Langbaurgh
is also the most geographically diverse of the Cleveland districts and
contains much of its rural portion. This helps to account for the fact
that it does not have a high concentration of wards in the Region's
worst 20 per cent on any of the indicators of deprivation — except
for unemployment. Across its length, from Eston to Loftus, wards
which do not feature as exceptional on other measures of deprivation
nevertheless experience unemployment rates sufficiently high to
place them in the Region's worst fifth. In all, exactly one half of
Cleveland's wards rank within the Region's worst quintile on
unemployment (as defined at the 1981 Census), the majority of these
in the extreme 10 per cent; whereas just over one-third of the Tyne
and Wear wards figure in the worst quintile, most of these in the less
extreme part of that range.

There is, of course, one major difference between unemployment
and the other three criteria of deprivation used in this study.
Unemployment directly reflects the social consequences of the

71

working of the economy. In these data the effects on employment of the decline of the Teesside and Hartlepool sub-regional economy, matched elsewhere in the Northern Region only in Consett, are clearly revealed. The other measures of deprivation have a different economic dimension, in that they represent aspects of consumption, whereas unemployment relates more immediately to production — and its contraction. South Tyneside heads the ranking on all these other three indicators, when the most deprived fifth of wards is considered. Apart from Middlesbrough, only Hartlepool of the Cleveland districts figures prominently on any of the indicators other than unemployment; whereas in contrast, all of the Tyne and Wear districts have sizeable concentrations of deprivation on each of these criteria. In Durham, Easington features prominently on the three measures other than unemployment, whilst in Derwentside and Wear Valley unemployment comes to the fore, coupled with over-crowding in Wear Valley and the lack of a car in Derwentside. One indicator which calls for special comment is that covering rented housing. Cleveland as a whole features less strongly on this than on any of the four measures of deprivation, but instead different areas come into the picture — Berwick, Blyth Valley and Sedgefield especially among districts which are not prominent on other criteria. It is also interesting to note that deprivation in the West Cumbrian districts of Allerdale and Copeland is most evident on this indicator and, secondly, on overcrowding — in other words, the two housing variables — rather than on unemployment or car ownership. Moreover, even though the proportion of deprived wards in Aller-dale and Copeland is small, Maryport, Workington and Whitehaven account for the majority of them.

Some features of non-urban deprivation remain to be discussed. It is commonly assumed that urban deprivation is more severe than rural deprivation, and that inner city deprivation in particular is more prevalent and a greater social problem than that encountered anywhere else. None of the evidence presented in this study so far would challenge this view. Certainly the areas in the Northern Region with the least deprivation are overwhelmingly rural. Admittedly, to a small extent it may be that deprivation in rural areas is concealed by the varied social composition of many wards, which will lessen the impact in statistics of any pockets of deprivation they may contain. Yet the Northern Region does contain two semi-rural, semi-urban belts in which deprivation is significant. West Cumbria and, even more, Durham both retain landscapes of industrial or, increasingly, declining and de-industrialised villages, typically either threatened by high unemployment or else already afflicted by it. The social uniformity of these strongly working-class localities ensures that pockets of marked deprivation are not concealed, and do emerge in ward figures. Wards like Craghead, Shotton, Old Trimdon, Thornley, Wheatley Hill and Tow Law, in Durham, or Cleator Moor South and Frizington in West Cumbria, do not register on our indicators of deprivation to the same extent as the deprived wards of the towns and cities of the Region; yet on certain criteria these wards are considerably deprived. This needs to be remembered when examining the connections between health and deprivation.

Finally, we conclude this chapter by extending our comparison of ward deprivation in order to contrast the Northern Region with Greater London. A current study of poverty and the London labour market (Townsend *et al.*, 1987) employs the same four indicators of deprivation as those used in the present study of 678 wards, in an analysis of 755 London wards. Unfortunately, it is not possible to compare overall deprivation in wards using the combined measure, but of the four individual indicators, three are directly comparable. On the criterion of unemployment, for example, all of the 25 wards (among the total of 1,433 in the two Regions) with the highest unemployment at the 1981 Census were in the Northern Region. On the criterion of non-owner occupation, the pattern was almost reversed, with just two of the 25 wards with highest levels of rented accommodation being in the North. The car possession indicator, on the other hand, was more evenly split at the most deprived end of the scale, with 14 of the 25 wards with lowest levels of car ownership being in the North. The fourth (overcrowding) indicator has been constructed in a slightly different manner in the two studies, making direct comparison impossible. Nevertheless, this is a measure on which the most adversely affected London wards experience higher levels of deprivation than the equivalent wards in the North. We do not intend to pursue this contrast more widely; but in the light of the studies by Jarman (1983, 1984, 1985) and the Department of the Environment (1983), referred to earlier (section 3.2), in which the outcome is the portrayal of deprivation as far greater in London than in the North, we would emphasise the disparity between indicators which reflect deprivation in the housing sphere, and the unemployment and non-car ownership indicators, which reflect lack of immediate income and other resources. In housing London clearly experiences the more pronounced deprivation; according to other basic criteria it is just as clearly the North which experiences greater deprivation.

6

The Link Between Health and Deprivation

So far we have concentrated attention on the separate distribution of poor health and deprivation in the Northern Region, and have identified the areas in which each is worst. More briefly, we have also identified the areas where the best health and least deprivation or greatest prosperity is to be found. In this chapter, regional inequalities in health are examined rather differently, applying quantile analysis to a large number of small areas. All 678 wards have been divided into quintile (20 per cent) bands, on the basis of the ward ranking on each of the health indicators in turn. The bands covering 10 per cent of wards at either extreme have also been picked out. This procedure will assist causal analysis, as well as highlight the full extent of the inequalities found in the Region. The second feature of this chapter is to bring together the independent sets of data on health and deprivation, in order to find how far patterns of deprivation are associated with patterns of health in the Region. As will become apparent, the correspondence between poor health and deprivation is extremely close.

6.1 THE RANGE OF VARIATION WITHIN THE REGION: OVERALL HEALTH

It is important to relate health to prosperity, and not only ill-health to deprivation. Concentration on the localities with the poorest health and greatest deprivation is essential if we are to identify the places — and by extension, the people — with the worst experience, so that such problems may be explained and perhaps rectified. However, there is a danger that if not placed in the context of the entire social structure, bad health and high levels of deprivation may

seem to be confined to certain areas and the people who live in then
This would be to spotlight part of the picture at the expense of th
whole: for by altering our viewpoint so that we look at the full range
of wards and the whole spectrum of health or deprivation, we begin
to understand the underlying structural causes of both health and ill-
health, as well as prosperity and deprivation. Inequality becomes the
centre-piece and explanatory theme of the study. It is this inequality
in health, and not just the bad health localities in isolation, which
invites description and explanation. Areas of bad health, like those
of great deprivation, account for only part of the geography of the
North, no less than of Britain as a whole. Areas of good as well as
bad health are both generated out of the inequalities which are
endemic in our society.

The range of variation in the Northern Region obtained by ranking wards on the Overall Health Index is presented in Table 6.1. The
10 per cent of wards with the worst overall health experience levels
of premature mortality and low birthweight more than twice as high,
and levels of permanent sickness and disability more than three
times as high, as the 10 per cent of wards with the best health.
Indeed, at the best end of the range, health levels as reflected by our
indicators compare favourably with almost any area in Britain: for
instance, the ward with the best health overall in Tyne and Wear (St
Mary's in North Tyneside) would rank alongside the best wards·in
Bristol (compare Townsend et al., 1984). A simple representation
of the evidence for each rank of wards is also given in Figure 6.1.
Displayed beneath the health information are the four main
indicators of material deprivation, together with other socio-
economic indicators selected from the 1981 Census. These reveal a
remarkably uniform and conclusive pattern, not only in the contrast
between the two extremes, but right across the whole range — for
the step-wise gradation of these indicators from one quintile to the
next very closely mirrors the gradation apparent on the health
criteria. The link between measures of health and socio-economic
measures reflecting deprivation could scarcely be more firmly
demonstrated. Unemployment is almost four times worse, overcrowding four-and-a-half times as likely, and car ownership and
owner occupation levels nearly three times lower, in the 10 per cent
of wards with the worst overall health, as compared with the best
10 per cent. At the same time, the less dramatic but nonetheless
noticeable contrast in health between the second and fourth quintile
bands finds a precise parallel in the social and economic sphere.

To what extent, however, is this pattern evident if we differentiate

Figure 6.1: The structure of inequality in the Northern Region: wards ranked on Overall Health Index

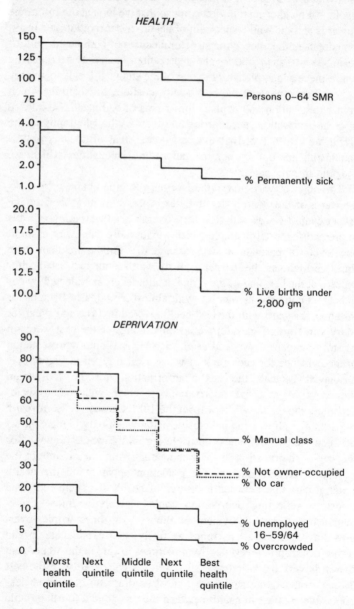

Table 6.1: Health and deprivation for ward groupings based on ranking of wards by Overall Health Index

	Worst health decile (68 wards)	Best health decile (68 wards)	Ratio Worst/Best	Worst health quintile (136 wards)	Next quintile (136 wards)	Middle quintile (134 wards)	Next quintile (136 wards)	Best health quintile (136 wards)
Persons 0–64 SMR	156.4	69.8	2.2	142.6	120.5	107.3	98.9	79.9
Residents 16+ permanently sick (%)	3.9	1.2	3.3	3.6	2.8	2.3	1.8	1.3
Live births under 2,800 gm (%)	18.7	8.4	2.2	17.9	15.1	14.1	12.7	10.1
Unemployed persons 16–59/64 (%)	22.8	5.9	3.9	20.2	15.6	11.4	9.1	6.3
Households not owner-occupied (%)	76.4	27.1	2.8	72.9	60.5	50.1	35.7	24.9
Households with no car (%)	67.4	23.4	2.9	64.3	55.4	45.5	35.9	23.6
Households with more persons than rooms (%)	6.5	1.4	4.6	5.9	4.2	3.2	2.2	1.5
Households with head in manual class (%)	80.6	37.8	2.1	77.9	71.8	63.0	52.0	40.8
Households without exclusive use of bath & WC (%)	3.4	2.4	1.4	3.4	4.3	3.2	3.0	2.0
Households with single parent family (%)	7.9	3.1	2.5	7.2	5.6	4.8	3.9	3.3
Unemployed persons 16–24 (%)	29.3	11.3	2.6	26.9	21.8	17.8	15.2	11.8
17-year olds not in full-time education (%)	83.9	47.6	1.8	82.7	77.0	71.1	62.2	49.3
Population	354,617	156,814		787,575	697,455	628,403	545,082	375,567

between the larger urban areas and the rural or smaller urban environment? Table 6.2 is based on a distinction between wards in urban areas containing a population over 20,000, and all remaining wards (described for convenience simply as non-urban: for details of this classification see Appendix 4). Only the extreme 10 per cent bands in the two categories are shown. The pattern in both cases conforms with that already described. However, the big difference between the urban and non-urban categories lies in the considerably higher mortality in the urban bloc, which extends right across the range of wards, and likewise in the higher levels of deprivation. Permanent sickness and low birthweight levels are only slightly higher in urban areas. At the same time, on two of the three health indicators the non-urban areas show a wider range of variation between the two extremes, particularly in the case of low birthweight. In contrast, the range of variation on the deprivation criteria is more pronounced in urban areas. In health terms, therefore, it is in its much worse mortality that the urban north must be differentiated from the rural parts of the Region. On permanent sickness and low birthweight the differences are much less clearcut.

Many readers will be interested in how our evidence applies to local authority areas and parliamentary constituencies. Accordingly, the next two tables set out the pertinent facts. Both sets of material confirm the close link between health and deprivation. The areas with poor health are those with marked deprivation, and vice versa. However, Table 6.3 also allows the value of an analysis of smaller areas such as wards to be recognised, because when data are aggregated for larger areas, a lot of telling evidence can become blurred. One example will make this point clear. Langbaurgh and South Tyneside both have identical mortality rates for premature deaths (SMRs of 119); but as Table 4.2 above showed, the range of variation within these two districts differs enormously, Langbaurgh having a very wide gap between its wards with highest and lowest mortality, and South Tyneside a much narrower gap. In such cases the district-level mortality ratio conceals more than it reveals.

Table 6.4 continues the same theme for the 36 parliamentary constituencies of the Northern Region. Tyne Bridge constituency is split equally between Newcastle and Gateshead. This constituency experiences the worst health on all three criteria, and the greatest deprivation on three of the four criteria. Its unemployment rate is second only to Middlesbrough as the highest in the entire Region. The most notable feature of its health experience is the mortality

Table 6.2: Health and deprivation for urban and non-urban ward groupings based on ranking of wards by Overall Health Index

	Urban wards			Non-urban wards		
	Worst health decile (34 wards)	Best health decile (34 wards)	Ratio Worst/Best	Worst health decile (34 wards)	Best health decile (34 wards)	Ratio Worst/Best
Persons 0–64 SMR	162.4	84.1	1.9	138.0	62.5	2.2
Residents 16+ permanently sick (%)	4.0	1.2	3.3	3.8	1.2	3.2
Live births under 2,800 gm (%)	19.4	10.6	1.8	17.6	6.8	2.6
Unemployed persons (%)	25.0	6.5	3.9	14.2	5.0	2.8
Households not owner-occupied (%)	77.2	13.8	5.6	66.4	31.5	2.1
Households with no car (%)	70.0	24.1	2.9	54.1	20.1	2.7
Households with > 1 person per room (%)	7.3	1.2	6.1	4.2	1.5	2.8
Population	207,128	178,067	—	111,760	58,225	—

Table 6.3: Health and deprivation in the local authorities of the Northern Region

Local authority	Persons 0–64 SMR	No. of deaths	% Perm. sick	No. Perm. sick	% Low weight births	No. Low weight births	% Un-employed	% Households with no car	% Households over-crowded	% Households not owner-occupied	% Class 4&5 households
Gateshead	125	2160	3.0	5011	15.3	1171	14.2	57.2	4.9	61.4	26.8
Newcastle upon Tyne	118	2609	2.7	5854	15.9	1641	14.5	58.8	4.6	61.1	23.5
North Tyneside	112	1879	2.4	3780	16.2	1111	12.6	52.9	3.3	55.1	22.1
South Tyneside	119	1636	2.7	3377	14.5	819	17.0	59.5	4.6	68.5	26.8
Sunderland	117	2643	2.9	6497	14.0	1755	16.9	54.6	4.6	62.0	24.5
Hartlepool	130	964	2.5	1774	16.5	642	18.2	52.3	4.2	49.4	31.6
Langbaurgh	119	1350	2.3	2571	13.2	798	16.1	41.9	3.7	39.9	27.3
Middlesbrough	130	1487	2.6	2921	15.6	1091	20.2	50.2	5.4	46.4	30.9
Stockton	117	1511	2.4	3097	16.6	1257	15.4	41.8	3.3	41.8	24.6
Allerdale	110	849	1.9	1361	14.7	495	10.9	37.9	2.8	46.4	26.2
Barrow-in-Furness	114	670	1.8	1010	14.1	394	9.8	45.7	2.7	28.3	22.6
Carlisle	104	836	1.9	1482	14.0	517	9.0	39.7	3.2	47.8	20.5
Copeland	114	645	1.9	1050	13.9	408	9.8	39.8	3.5	55.1	30.2
Eden	96	326	1.5	505	13.4	178	6.2	26.0	2.1	43.5	20.6
South Lakeland	93	692	1.4	996	11.7	318	5.6	28.7	1.7	36.3	17.0
Chester-le-Street	113	445	2.7	1069	14.1	293	11.0	41.9	2.9	47.6	21.0
Darlington	114	886	2.0	1452	15.3	561	10.7	44.8	2.9	34.5	22.6
Derwentside	117	841	3.3	2278	14.4	465	22.4	50.8	3.4	50.7	27.6
Durham	110	693	2.7	1706	13.8	415	9.3	42.7	3.1	52.7	23.2
Easington	122	987	3.8	2909	15.9	618	12.3	56.7	4.4	69.6	29.2
Sedgefield	116	845	2.9	2013	15.6	568	12.8	48.1	3.3	61.5	32.1
Teesdale	84	169	2.1	394	16.6	124	8.4	33.3	2.6	43.8	25.7

Wear Valley	122	641	3.5	1733	15.2	345	15.4	49.1	4.7	49.4	28.9
Alnwick	93	208	2.0	430	13.8	141	8.7	38.8	3.1	59.8	26.5
Berwick upon Tweed	113	232	1.8	353	13.6	112	8.6	40.1	3.1	65.3	28.9
Blyth Valley	106	581	1.9	1107	13.2	453	10.5	41.9	2.4	50.7	23.0
Castle Morpeth	92	360	1.7	633	11.9	168	5.7	29.3	2.6	45.6	16.4
Tynedale	92	393	1.9	782	11.4	208	6.5	34.4	2.7	47.0	21.5
Wansbeck	115	604	2.8	1348	14.7	326	9.8	51.4	3.2	60.9	25.0
Northern Region	115	28,142	2.5	59,493	14.8	17,392	13.5	48.3	3.8	52.9	25.2
England and Wales	100	—	1.8	—	NAᵃ	—	9.8	38.5	3.4	42.2	21.7

Note: a. England and Wales data for live births under 2,800 gm are not available. Over the period 1982–4 the proportion of live births under 2,500 gm was 6.5 per cent in the Northern Region and 6.7 per cent in England and Wales.
Additional sources: OPCS, *1981 Census National Reports*; OPCS Monitors DH3 84/7, 85/1, 85/5.

Table 6.4: Health and deprivation in the parliamentary constituencies of the Northern Region

Parliamentary constituency	Health indicators			% unemployed 16–59/64	Deprivation indicators		
	Persons 0–64 SMR	% residents 16+ permanently sick	% live births under 2,800 gm		% households over-crowded	% households with no car	% households not owner-occupied
Barrow and Furness	113	1.7	13.8	9.2	2.6	42.8	28.9
Berwick upon Tweed	101	2.0	13.5	8.5	3.3	39.3	62.7
Bishop Auckland	113	2.8	15.9	12.9	4.0	45.3	55.4
Blaydon	111	2.9	13.0	10.9	3.1	47.8	47.0
Blyth Valley	106	1.9	13.2	10.5	2.4	41.9	50.7
Carlisle	109	2.1	14.7	9.8	3.7	46.9	50.8
Copeland	114	1.9	13.9	9.8	3.5	39.9	55.1
Darlington	117	2.0	15.6	11.4	3.1	47.9	35.8
Durham, City of	110	2.7	13.8	9.3	3.1	42.7	52.7
Durham North	113	3.2	14.9	15.1	3.2	47.3	49.8
Durham North-West	118	3.1	13.4	20.3	3.7	47.6	49.6
Easington	119	3.7	15.6	12.0	4.6	56.8	69.8
Gateshead East	125	2.9	16.0	15.3	6.0	60.0	69.5
Hartlepool	130	2.5	16.5	18.2	4.2	52.3	49.4
Hexham	91	1.8	11.5	5.8	2.3	30.1	43.5
Houghton and Washington	114	2.9	13.9	13.1	3.4	47.9	64.7
Jarrow	115	2.8	14.2	17.5	4.9	57.6	71.9
Langbaurgh	110	2.1	12.6	14.3	3.3	34.7	37.5
Middlesbrough	141	3.0	16.6	23.6	6.5	60.0	51.0

Newcastle upon Tyne Central	118	15.3	2.5	12.7	3.7	54.2	55.9
Newcastle upon Tyne East	121	15.0	2.9	15.5	4.8	67.3	66.8
Newcastle upon Tyne North	101	14.7	2.4	11.4	3.5	47.5	54.4
Penrith and the Border	99	13.5	1.6	6.7	2.2	25.2	41.8
Redcar	127	14.4	2.5	18.6	4.4	48.1	46.8
Sedgefield	118	15.6	3.1	12.0	3.0	45.8	54.2
South Shields	123	14.8	2.6	16.5	4.2	61.4	65.0
Stockton North	121	17.1	2.8	17.6	3.6	48.2	50.7
Stockton South	113	15.6	2.0	12.9	3.0	34.3	29.2
Sunderland North	119	14.2	2.9	20.3	5.9	61.6	61.1
Sunderland South	119	14.0	3.0	17.4	4.3	53.8	60.4
Tyne Bridge	153	18.9	3.7	21.5	7.2	72.8	74.0
Tynemouth	106	15.3	2.1	12.1	2.9	49.3	44.9
Wallsend	118	16.9	2.8	13.0	3.6	56.3	64.8
Wansbeck	111	14.0	2.5	8.9	3.1	47.8	57.4
Westmorland & Lonsdale	89	11.6	1.5	5.5	1.7	28.4	37.7
Workington	111	14.5	1.9	11.9	2.9	40.4	47.8
Northern Region	115	14.8	2.5	13.5	3.8	48.3	52.9

rate: a constituency-wide SMR of 153 is dramatic testimony to the severity of its levels of ill-health.

6.2 PREMATURE MORTALITY

The pattern of inequality which we have described can be replicated if wards are ranked on any one of the health indicators. In this section, however, we will give primary attention to mortality, because a more detailed analysis can be given than in either of the other instances of low birthweight and adult chronic sickness. Some exposition of the latter will be found in Appendix 5 (Tables A5.1 and A5.2). When the Northern Region's 678 wards are ranked according to number of deaths relative to population aged under 65 (i.e. 0–64 SMR), the variation is very large. Those 10 per cent of wards with highest premature mortality experience levels of death almost three times worse than those at the other extreme (the 10 per cent with lowest mortality). Let us consider what this would mean if translated into numbers of deaths. Had the 10 per cent of wards with highest mortality experienced the mortality of the 10 per cent of wards at the opposite extreme, then the total number of people dying under the age of 65 over the three years covered would have been 1,524, instead of the 4,319 deaths which actually occurred. In other words, by the yardstick of the wards with the lowest mortality in the Region, there were 930 'excess' deaths *each year* in the wards with highest mortality. The evidence for the extreme 10 per cent bands is presented in Table 6.5, alongside a breakdown of SMRs for both sexes separately and for different age-groups. Data covering the full range of wards in quintile bands is to be found in Appendix 5 (Table A5.3).

The pattern is complex. Firstly, the pattern for specific sex and age bands closely reflects the overall step-wise gradient of the main (0–64) mortality variable (only the death rate for male children under 15 departs slightly from this gradient in the middle ranges of the distribution). Secondly, although standardised death rates for age-groups under 65 in the 10 per cent of wards with highest mortality are all at least twice as high as the 10 per cent with lowest mortality, the range of variation is greatest and the relative death rates highest at ages 45–64 for both sexes. The female rate at these ages is the highest figure of all (with an SMR of 175). Only at ages 65–74 does the range of variation narrow. These findings provide a pattern of inequality demanding explanation. They show that

Table 6.5: Health and deprivation for ward groupings based on ranking of wards by persons 0–64 SMR

	Worst mortality decile (68 wards)	Best mortality decile (68 wards)	Ratio Worst/Best
Persons 0–64 SMR	165.2 (4319)	58.3 (659)	2.8
Live births under 2,800 gm (%)	17.7	11.1	1.6
Residents 16+ permanently sick (%)	3.5	1.4	2.5
Infant mortality rate (deaths under 1 year per 1,000 live births)	13.4 (213)	8.0 (34)	1.7
Male 0–14 SMR	153.6 (186)	63.5 (29)	2.4
Female 0–14 SMR	139.8 (124)	49.7 (16)	2.8
Male 15–44 SMR	153.0 (351)	62.4 (62)	2.5
Female 15–44 SMR	141.4 (172)	65.0 (38)	2.2
Male 45–64 SMR	165.1 (2166)	55.8 (315)	3.0
Female 45–64 SMR	174.9 (1320)	60.0 (199)	2.9
Male 65–74 SMR	131.2 (2122)	89.8 (689)	1.5
Female 65–74 SMR	131.6 (1452)	92.1 (475)	1.4
Unemployed persons (%)	22.0	5.8	3.8
Households not owner-occupied (%)	72.1	30.5	2.4
Households with no car (%)	66.1	24.2	2.7
Households with more persons than rooms (%)	6.5	1.5	4.3

Note: Actual number of deaths in parentheses.

inequality in mortality in the North is actually greatest in the two decades leading up to retirement, before narrowing considerably thereafter. This pattern has interest in relation to the *national* evidence on social differentials in mortality at different ages, which is examined in Chapter 10. It seems that the pattern of inequality in the North is somewhat different from the national pattern. Before the age of 45 the ratio of combined Classes IV and V to combined Classes I and II is approximately the same as for the country as a whole: thereafter it is larger.

In relation to England and Wales as a whole, it is apparent that even in the middle ranges of the regional distribution mortality is relatively worse over the age of 45 than it is under 45. Thus, SMRs relating to deaths under 45 in the middle quintile are all beneath 100 for both sexes, and only the two worst quintiles exceed the national average (see Appendix 5, Table A5.3). However, this is not the case for the 45–64 age-group, where the middle quintile SMRs for both sexes are by some margin greater than the England and Wales average. This trend is also evident when the 65–74 age-group is considered, for in this case even the second best quintile has death rates exceeding the national average. This evidence helps to suggest that not only is inequality in mortality within the Region widest in the two decades up to the age of 65, but also that it is in this age range that mortality is highest in relation to England and Wales. Furthermore, when we compare mortality in turn with indicators of deprivation, class and other social factors, the same consistent pattern of variation is revealed. Higher premature mortality at every quintile step corresponds with higher unemployment, greater over-crowding and lower levels of car ownership and owner occupation. These appear, therefore, as different dimensions of a common social experience.

The analysis of mortality can be taken further by examining specific causes of death (Table 6.6). In this table, based on the headings used in the International Classification of Diseases (ICD), we have selected for illustration the three most common classes of death in Britain today: all cancers combined (neoplasms); circulatory system diseases, which includes heart attack and stroke; and respiratory system diseases. We have also extracted from the overall cancer picture three more specific groups: lung cancers, breast cancer and cancers of the digestive organs, which between them acount for approximately two out of every three cancer deaths. In addition, we have added SMRs for accidents, poisoning and violence, together with a crude rate for suicides and self-inflicted

Table 6.6: Mortality by cause of death. SMRs for deaths between 0 and 64 for ward groupings based on ranking of wards by persons 0–64 SMRs (actual numbers of deaths in parentheses)

Cause and sex		Worst mortality decile (68 wards)		Best mortality decile (68 wards)		Ratio Worst/Best
All causes	M	162.7	(2703)	57.2	(406)	2.8
	F	167.6	(1616)	60.0	(253)	2.8
All neoplasms (ICD 140–239)	M	172.1	(770)	60.7	(117)	2.8
	F	145.0	(576)	68.2	(121)	2.1
Malignant neoplasms of trachea, bronchus and lung (ICD 162)	M	217.3	(361)	49.9	(36)	4.4
	F	244.1	(146)	53.2	(14)	4.6
Malignant neoplasms of digestive organs and peritoneum (ICD 150–159)	M	161.1	(203)	60.3	(33)	2.7
	F	158.7	(120)	59.0	(20)	2.7
Malignant neoplasms of female breast (ICD 174)		99.4	(108)	89.1	(44)	1.1
Diseases of circulatory system (ICD 390–459)	M	159.4	(1147)	61.1	(191)	2.6
	F	210.2	(564)	53.0	(63)	4.0
Diseases of respiratory system (ICD 460–519)	M	199.5	(229)	37.6	(18)	5.3
	F	229.4	(159)	41.5	(12)	5.5
Accidents, poisonings and violence (ICD E800–999)	M	148.8	(260)	59.7	(42)	2.5
	F	131.6	(90)	69.9	(20)	1.9
Suicide and self-inflicted injury (ICD E950–E959): deaths between 15 and 64 per 100,000 population	M	57.8	(62)	29.2	(13)	2.0
	F	25.9	(27)	15.6	(7)	1.7
'Avoidable' deaths[a]	M	167	(287)	52	(38)	3.2
	F	185	(291)	39	(27)	4.7
Population of Ward Grouping		326,850		138,813		—

Note: a. This category includes diseases for which mortality is largely avoidable given appropriate medical intervention (References 1, 2, 3 below): Tuberculosis (010–018, 137), Malignant neoplasm of cervix uteri (180), Hodgkin's disease (201), Chronic rheumatic heart disease (393–398), Hypertensive disease (401–405), Cerebrovascular disease (430–438), Appendicitis (540–543), Cholelithiasis and cholecystitis (574–575.1), Pneumonia and bronchitis (480–486, 490), Asthma (493), Acute respiratory disease (460–466, 470–474), Abdominal hernia (550–553), Bacterial infections (004, 037, 320–322, 382–384, 390–392, 680–686, 711, 730), Maternal deaths (630–678), Deficiency anaemias (280–281).
References:
   1. Charlton, J.R.H., Hartley, R.M., Silver, R. and Holland, W.W. (1983).
   2. Charlton, J.R.H., Bauer, R. and Lakhani, A. (1984).
   3. Charlton, J.R.H. and Velez, R. (1986).

injury. Finally, we have compared all 'medically avoidable' deaths, a category which covers a number of common and rare causes sharing, according to prevailing medical opinion, the characteristic of being preventable, given timely and appropriate medical intervention. Further data on specific avoidable deaths and area variations in all avoidable deaths are given in Appendix 5 (Tables A5.4 and A5.5).

With the sole exception of breast cancer, where the SMRs are close to or slightly better than the England and Wales average across the spectrum of wards, all of the causes highlighted demonstrate considerable inequality between the two extremes, and the by now familiar pattern of variation from one quintile band to the next. In other words, the same consistent configuration is apparent. The inequality is widest with respiratory deaths, where the SMRs for both sexes in the worst 10 per cent of wards are more than five times higher than in the best 10 per cent; but the ratio is also more than 4:1 in the case of lung cancer for both sexes, and medically avoidable deaths in women, and close to 4:1 for female deaths from circulatory causes. The ratio is also more than 3:1 for medically avoidable deaths among men. Leaving aside breast cancer, only female deaths due to accidents, etc., exhibit a pattern of inequality where the ratio is less than 2:1.

These results reflect national inequalities by causes and by class (OPCS, 1978; Townsend and Davidson, 1982, pp. 54–5). Moreover, our quite different approach highlights the inequalities without raising the particular methodological problems now frequently attributed to occupational class categories. It also depicts the regional pattern in relation to the national average, and demonstrates once more how pronounced these mortality differentials are. This is a topic to which we shall return.

6.3 LIFE IN THE POOREST WARDS

What does deprivation mean for the areas with poor health which we have described? There have recently been several accounts of what inequality in Britain today means for those who are poorest, in explicit recognition of the severity of the present economic recession and its social consequences. Among the best examples are those by Campbell (1984) and Seabrook (1985), dovetailing the individual experience of being poor, as expressed through the words of the poor themselves, with documentation of the material conditions within which these experiences take place. We take a slightly different path here, concentrating on place rather than individual people, and on the outward signs of an enduring and deeply embedded inequality, rather than on personal testimony.

Visual images of poverty are controversial but influential, for popular conceptions of what poverty means tenaciously persist in making the recollections of an earlier period the yardstick by which to judge the present. Yet despite disagreement over the nature of poverty, few people find it hard to assess the relative affluence or deprivation of different communities. Material well-being has its public and visible aspect, and people are generally attuned not only to the grosser disparities but also to the nuances of much diminished or more local markers of wealth and living standards. This is in obvious contrast with differences in health between one locality and another, which remain scarcely visible in any literal sense, and can usually only be inferred in an approximate way from the affluence or deprivation of the localities in question.

We will outline some of the physical and material characteristics which differentiate in economic terms some of Easington's villages and the northern end of Whitley Bay. The wards of Wheatley Hill, Thornley, Shotton and Wingate make up a group of villages in the south-west of Easington District. All experience health which is among the very worst in the Region, using the criterion of overall health which we have adopted. As communities they share many common characteristics. Although the area remains largely rural, in the sense that these are villages which are surrounded by agricultural land, the villages are industrial in nature, more akin to very small towns in their layout, and owe either their existence or their expansion to coal. Today, however, they are pit villages without pits, all four pits in these villages having been closed by the early 1970s; and since 1981, two of the three remaining pits nearby have also closed, leaving Easington's mine alone in the vicinity.

Close together, so that no more than a mile or two of open countryside intervenes as one passes from one village to the next, all four are large enough to support small high streets, and not just an isolated village shop. However, these are scarcely thriving high streets, and reveal in the range of goods that are available something of the poor economic circumstances of perhaps the majority of the population. Many shops have been forced to close, nowhere suffering more than Wingate, once the hub of West Easington and almost a small town. Housing varies in quality, but new building is continuing to take place on a small scale; and from appearances the housing in general betrays few of the obvious signs of physical deterioration or dereliction of the bleakest and most deprived inner city areas or the barren post-war estates built around the urban fringe.

It is in the environment beyond the home that the deprivation facing these communities is most readily sensed: not just in the sparse shops, but in the paucity of other services and facilities which might be expected in a more affluent locality. Above all, the unnaturally neat contours of ground that has been landscaped in the recent past are a potent reminder of the pits which once occupied the scene and have now disappeared, evoking Seabrook's vivid metaphor for a process which has been occurring in many parts of the country:

> A sustained effort has been made, it seems, to wipe out the traces of the industrial revolution . . . The scars of that epic ugliness have been healed . . . In all the industrial districts, they have been burying the remains. It has the grandeur of the careful concealment of some epic crime (1985, p. 27).

It might be a different matter if new opportunities for work had replaced the old, but they have not, either in these villages themselves or in Peterlee. In comparison with the areas in the north-east where unemployment was highest in 1981, rates in Easington suggested a markedly less desperate situation. However, not only have matters worsened since then; even in 1981 the much higher rates of unemployment in the 16–24 age-group indicated the coming trend and the absence of prospects for the rising generation, as coal ceased to offer a reliable hope for more than a small number.

The inevitable consequences of disappearing livelihoods are increasing deprivation and the demographic distortion which comes from the young being forced to move away. These are problems which pose severe threats to small and relatively isolated communities, despite their close-knit character and deep sense of identity. Now these villages are not alone in their predicament: elsewhere in County Durham there are similar pit villages confronting comparable deprivation, especially in Wear Valley, Derwentside and Sedgefield. Some also experience health as bad as that occurring in many parts of Easington, thereby placing them among the very worst in the Region. However, where Easington stands out is in its consistently poor health, on all three of our chosen criteria and across an almost continuous band of wards. The four villages of Wheatley Hill, Thornley, Shotton and Wingate epitomise this unenviable condition in an extreme form.

By way of a complete contrast, the northern part of Whitley Bay is an area which enjoys a health record as good as anywhere in Tyne and Wear and among the best in the North. It is also among the most affluent or least deprived parts of the North. The wards of St Mary's and Monkseaton, in North Tyneside, have somewhat different characters but share a similar class composition. Monkseaton contains much of the older, middle-class residential part of Whitley Bay, whereas the larger part of St Mary's consists of newer housing estates for owner occupiers in higher income brackets. Monkseaton therefore has a more established character than St Mary's, but not necessarily a lower turnover of population. The most distinctive feature of these two wards is not that they contain pockets of great affluence: other parts of the Tyneside commuter belt are probably better examples in that respect. Rather, it is the even spread of comparatively well-off households which distinguishes this area. Much good quality housing, a level of public transport provision which bears no comparison with the Easington villages, a number of shopping centres with a wide range of shops and goods, wide streets, and plenty of open spaces with a variety of leisure facilities for those who can afford them: these are some of the signs of a locality which attracts those who are better-off, and continues to thrive, even during such a severe recession as the present one. Above all, Whitley Bay has the sea. So also does Easington. But the seaside setting of sandy beaches which has given Whitley Bay its resort reputation is a very far cry from the scarred and often heavily polluted coastline, blackened in places with coal waste, of even the rural parts of Easington. Unemployment — and more particularly youth unemployment — has not bypassed St Mary's and Monkseaton. However, it has started rising from an inevitably far lower baseline, and is growing at a slower rate, than in the hard-hit areas. It remains atypically low in regional terms, though in national terms it is almost certainly higher than in areas of comparable social composition in southern towns or cities. In addition, this is an area in which a relatively high proportion of children postpone their entry into the labour market by remaining at school to the age of 17 and beyond, and then by pursuing higher education options.

Part Three:

Explanation

7

Occupational Class and
the Explanation of Health Inequalities

In describing present inequalities in health in the Northern Region, we have concentrated so far on two matters: the unequal geographical distribution of poor health, and the considerable variation between small areas with the best and worst health. However, populations are not randomly located. Some areas are much more desirable than others in which to live, and localities differ considerably in their class composition. Underlying, therefore, but not entirely explaining, area differences in health are class differences. How far do these explain the area differences which have been noted? In the last chapter a strong correlation was demonstrated between health indices and various measures of material deprivation, as well as the proportion of households with a manual class 'head'. In this chapter, the connection between class and health in the North will be examined in greater detail, using data on occupations derived from death and birth registrations. Following the references in Chapter 1, we will introduce the Registrar General's model of class.

7.1 THE TREATMENT OF CLASS

Over the years since its inception, the Registrar General's method of constructing a model of the social class structure of British society by the grading of occupations has been widely used, but it has also been criticised. The complex phenomenon of social class is reduced to an occupational classification alone, and even this does not have secure and clearly agreed theoretical foundations (Black Report, 1980, pp. 13–20). It is preferable, therefore, to speak of 'occupational class', recognising this as a crude surrogate for a more general conception of class (see, for example, Townsend, 1979, pp. 369–71; Black Report, 1980, p. 18): yet even as an occupational classification it is ambiguous. We mean not only that the criterion for classifying jobs has changed from general standing in the community to a grouping of people with similar levels of occupational skill (OPCS, 1970, 1980), but that both of these notions have continued to be problematic, if not contentious. In addition, the classification is not applied consistently to women, so that empirical analysis of female occupational class patterns is very difficult (see, for example, Goldthorpe, 1983, 1984; Heath and Britten, 1984; Stanworth, 1984). More generally, this model perpetuates an influential but misleading idea that society consists of five or six ranks ordered in a single, continuous hierarchy (Szreter, 1984, pp. 538–40). These points will be developed in greater detail in Chapter 10, where the latest national evidence is reported and assessed.

As a rough and ready research tool, the Registrar General's operational classification is worth maintaining because more sophisticated approaches (like that of Goldthorpe and his colleagues) do not appear to produce results which are in practice markedly different, and because it has the convenience of widespread use. The criticisms of the traditional method of representing social class made in the Black Report were made more to encourage the development of refined methods of scientific description than to impugn either the concept of social class or its approximate measurement by means of occupational status. One problem about the Decennial Supplement of 1986 (see OPCS, 1986; and below, Chapter 9) is that the relatively minor technical difficulties of adjusting classifications from decade to decade are allowed to obscure more important questions of the scientific scale and trends in mortality of the difference between the classes. Major elements of society's structure must not be lost sight of when the less major elements come to be examined.

7.2 CLASS GRADIENTS IN MORTALITY AND LOW BIRTHWEIGHT

We turn to present data on occupational class for the 678 wards in the North of England. Regrettably, most attention has to be given to male deaths, and specifically economically active men (aged 16–64). As already noted, records of women's occupations at death registration are notoriously incomplete or unreliable and it is

Table 7.1: Crude death rates (per 1,000 population) by Occupational Class for economically active men aged 16–64 in the Northern Region. Ward groupings (worst and best) based on ranking or wards by persons 0–64 SMR

Occupational class	Northern Region (all 678 wards)		Worst 20% (136 wards)		Best 20% (136 wards)	
	Annual Rate	Deaths 1982–3	Annual Rate	Deaths 1982–3	Annual Rate	Deaths 1982–3
I	2.7	(190)	3.0	(23)	2.1	(32)
II	3.9	(1122)	5.4	(192)	2.6	(141)
IIIN	4.3	(706)	5.5	(154)	2.7	(57)
IIIM	4.9	(3416)	6.2	(1073)	2.9	(180)
IV	6.4	(1891)	7.9	(643)	3.3	(98)
V	9.0	(1246)	10.5	(523)	4.8	(40)
I + II	3.7	(1312)	5.0	(215)	2.5	(173)
IV + V	7.2	(3137)	8.9	(1166)	3.7	(138)

Note: Men who retired before age 64 are excluded.

difficult to analyse women's mortality by their own occupational class. Table 7.1 presents crude death rates for men aged 16–64 for the Registrar General's classes covering the whole Northern Region and also the rates for the best and worst 20 per cent of wards (as ranked on the main mortality variable). The data are imperfect: crude, rather than age-standardised, death rates for occupational classes have had to be used. However, the imperfections have been lessened, insofar as the best and worst 20 per cent of wards have been defined initially on the basis of age-standardised mortality. The table illustrates the advantages of bringing together the two different methods of identifying health inequalities by class and by area.

The overall regional pattern revealed here broadly conforms with existing knowledge of national occupational class mortality (see Chapter 10): for example, men in combined Classes IV and V are subject to death rates which are nearly twice as high as combined Class I and II. Generally speaking, area mortality rates are correlated with class, in the sense that high rates are associated with relatively high proportions of the poorer manual classes in those areas, and vice versa. However, the correlation is far from complete or uniform, as our evidence will go on to show.

One striking feature of Table 7.1 is the difference between classes in the two bands of wards at opposite extremes of health. Combined Classes IV and V in the wards with lowest mortality have a lower death rate than combined Classes I and II in the band of wards with highest mortality. Class V on its own in the band with best health has lower mortality than all classes except Class I in the band with worst health. However, these deaths represent a very small proportion indeed of Class V deaths in the whole Region, and this paradoxical finding must therefore, not be allowed to overshadow the principal relationship between poorer occupational class and poorer health. There are also fluctuations in numbers of deaths from year to year, and despite adding together total deaths for two years, it is desirable in the case of the smallest wards to consider the experience for a longer span.

Presentation of the two bands each of 136 wards in Table 7.1 also helps to bring out the fact that there are divergent trends. Whereas the class gradient rises steeply in the wards with highest mortality, the rise in the wards with lowest mortality is much more gradual. Furthermore, to express the gap between the occupational class groups at their most extreme, the reader can see that the ratio of Class V in the band of wards with high mortality to Class I in the band with low mortality is no less than 5:1. Although this contrasts with the experience of relatively small clusters of people, it is one of the best measures of the full extent of inequality among social groups within the Region.

How can such contrasting outcomes begin to be explained? There are different possibilities. Firstly, the relatively good quality of climate, water, soil, air, location, transport and housing in some wards may contribute to the improved health experience of all occupational classes living in those wards. However, in calling attention to these different features of location, it is frustrating to have to report that there are insufficient means available at present to pin down which are more important for health than others. All we can confirm is the apparent advantage of some locations, especially those with the highest percentages of the population in occupational Classes I and II. We would echo Skrimshire's (1978) observation, arising out of a comparative study of health in three different council estates, that 'a working-class person is at a greater disadvantage if he lives in a predominantly working-class area than if he lives in a socially mixed area'. Localities have social and economic features which are of collective advantage or disadvantage and which appear to influence health decisively.

There is a second possibility. The health difference between identical classes living in different sets of wards may be due to a very different mix of the occupations of people in those classes. The possible importance of this lies in the fact that the mortality risk of specific occupations within the same class varies considerably (see, for example, Jones and Cameron, 1984, p. 43). However, the variation may itself reflect a difference of locality or environment as well as of occupation. In this case, for instance, we know that the two sets of wards at either end of the health spectrum contain a very different balance of urban and rural wards. This has a direct bearing on manual class patterns of mortality, partly because those in manual classes tend to work closer to home than people in Classes I and II. It is likely, therefore, that the occupations making up Classes III, IV and V in urban and rural wards will be very different, though probably not as different for the occupations making up the non-manual classes.

There are, of course, other possible explanations for the results shown in the table. The working conditions of people in similar occupations who live in different areas might have different implications for health. Again, the length of residence in given areas of people in identical occupational classes might be short or long; the good or poor health of some of them may be attributable to residence for many years elsewhere. Evidently, geographical factors are not easy to disentangle from strictly occupational factors in interpreting the results in Table 7.1. The results are striking enough to justify further analysis. The challenge to the sciences is not simply one which concerns the poorer health experiences of the manual classes. Our evidence shows how much greater is the mortality risk faced by Classes I and II in the 'worst' than in the 'best' set of wards. The figures suggest why it is important to come back to the impact of that wider set of influences which shape the whole living environment and social experience of people living in different kinds of areas. We shall return to this theme in the next chapter. This is plainly a different scientific path from one based on 'specific aetiology'. For the present it is sufficient just to draw attention to the non-occupational considerations which underlie analysis of health and mortality in the different occupational classes.

Occupational class mortality in the two extreme bands of 20 per cent of wards can also be examined in relation to major causes of death. Table 7.2 presents a four-way comparison between non-manual and manual classes in wards of high and low mortality. There are no striking differences in the distribution of the main causes, other than an indication that among manual class men in the 20 per cent of wards with highest mortality, lung cancer and respiratory causes account for twice as large a proportion of all deaths as among non-manual class men in the 20 per cent of wards

99

Table 7.2: Crude death rates (per 1,000 population) by Occupational Class (non-manual and manual) and cause of death for economically active men aged 16–64 in the Northern Region. Worst and best quintile of wards ranked on persons 0–64 SMR

Occupational Class (non-manual and manual) and cause of death	Worst 20% (136 wards)			Best 20% (136 wards)		
	Annual rate	Deaths 1982–83	Per cent of all causes	Annual rate	Deaths 1982–83	Per cent of all causes
Non-manual Classes (I, II, IIIN)						
All causes	5.2	369	100.0	2.6	230	100.0
Neoplasms (ICD 140–239)	1.5	106	28.7	0.7	65	28.3
Malignant neoplasms of digestive system (ICD 150–159)	0.5	36	9.7	0.2	18	7.8
Malignant neoplasms of trachea, bronchus and lung (ICD 162)	0.5	34	9.2	0.2	17	7.4
Diseases of circulatory system (ICD 390–459)	2.6	183	49.6	1.3	121	52.6
Diseases of respiratory system (ICD 460–519)	0.2	17	4.6	0.1	7	3.0
Accidents and violence (ICD E800–E999)	0.5	33	8.9	0.3	25	10.9
Manual Classes (IIIM, IV, V)						
All causes	7.3	2239	100.0	3.2	318	100.0
Neoplasms (ICD 140–239)	2.3	705	31.5	0.9	93	29.2
Malignant neoplasms of digestive system (ICD 150–159)	0.6	196	8.7	0.3	30	9.4
Malignant neoplasms of trachea, bronchus and lung (ICD 162)	1.0	304	13.6	0.3	33	10.4
Diseases of circulatory system (ICD 390–459)	3.3	1015	45.3	1.6	158	49.7
Diseases of respiratory system (ICD 460–519)	0.5	160	7.1	0.1	12	3.8
Accidents and violence (ICD E800–E999)	0.6	191	8.5	0.4	43	13.5

Note: Men who retired before age 65 are excluded.

with lowest mortality. This apart, men of manual class in the 'worst' bands of wards simply die more frequently from all causes than their counterparters in the other categories.

The available data on low birthweight and occupational class (based on the class of the father except where the mother lives apart) can be subjected to a similar kind of analysis, with similar results (Table 7.3). The region's wards have been divided into the 50 per cent with the highest and the 50 per cent with the lowest incidence of low birthweight babies (as ranked on the basis of the birthweight indicator). This proportion has been used because only 10 per cent of births are selected for occupation coding: numbers are therefore too small for a reliable analysis using the two extreme bands of 20 per cent of wards. Even so, the figures show that the incidence of low-weight births is less among the manual classes combined in the 50 per cent of wards with best health, than among the non-manual classes combined in the 50 per cent of wards with worst health. Moreover, a problem that we recognised in discussing occupational class mortality among men — that of the different risks attached to specific occupations grouped within the same class — does not arise in the analysis of low birthweight patterns by class. Various factors are undoubtedly involved, but the disparity between the experience of each occupational class in the two sets of wards is not in any sense a by-product of the mode of occupational classification. Rather, we are once again confronted with the influence of locality and the wider socio-economic environment on health.

7.3 EXCESS MORTALITY AND OCCUPATIONAL CLASS

The relationship between mortality and occupational class allows different ideas of 'excess' mortality (referred to already in Chapter 6) to be developed. We have seen that there are sharp differences between groups of wards ranked according to the mortality of people under 65 years of age. It is of course possible to define 'excess' mortality as mortality additional to that arising in Class I or Classes I and II which occurs in other classes. That has been done in previous health studies for illustrative purposes (e.g. Black Report, 1980, p. 3); but the idea can be applied in other ways to assist causal analysis. Thus, for example, we decided to ask how much of the mortality in the 10 or 20 per cent of wards with the highest death rates might be attributed to the occupational class structure of that group of wards, and how much remained unaccounted for, or

Table 7.3: Low birthweight by Occupational Class in the Northern Region. Ward groupings based on ranking of wards by low birthweight (proportion of live births under 2,800 gm). 10% sample

Occupational Class	Northern Region (All 678 wards)		Worst 50% (339 wards)		Best 50% (339 wards)	
	Live births under 2,800 gm		Live births under 2,800 gm		Live births under 2,800 gm	
	%	Number	%	Number	%	Number
I	11.1	62	12.3	29	10.2	33
II	11.6	185	13.3	93	10.2	92
IIIN	13.0	152	15.1	91	10.8	61
IIIM	14.6	632	15.6	406	13.0	226
IV	15.7	311	18.1	225	11.6	86
V	17.4	229	18.7	182	13.6	47
I + II	11.5	247	13.0	122	10.2	125
IV + V	16.4	540	18.4	407	12.2	133
Total number of live births	119,248		70,276		48,972	
Total number of live births for which social class known	11,944		7041		4903	

'excess', even after adjusting for the class structure. This is the question which we shall endeavour to answer.

This part of the analysis is presented for both sexes, and not just for men of employment age. Nonetheless, male deaths between 15 and 64 necessarily provide the principal data, for, as we have mentioned previously, it is only in relation to the deaths of men that the occupational class data are sufficiently complete to permit reasonably assured investigation. We have therefore needed to make the crude, but perhaps acceptable assumption that the female class structure in wards mirrors the male class structure. In Figure 7.1, SMRs predicted on the basis of the class composition of wards in each band of 20 per cent of wards and in the two extreme 10 per cent bands in the Region are contrasted with the actual (that is, the conventional, age-standardised) SMRs. This brings out graphically, the extent to which the actual mortality gradient is much steeper, right across the range, than would be predicted on the basis of national class mortality patterns alone. The predicted gradient is such that mortality in the worst 10 per cent of wards may be expected to be 1.3 times greater than in the most fortunate 10 per cent of wards. In reality, the former bloc experiences mortality 2.8 times higher than in the latter. At the same time, it is significant that only in the band of 10 per cent of wards with lowest mortality is the predicted SMR below the national average (i.e. 100): otherwise, right across the range, premature mortality in the North is predicted on the basis of class to be above the national average.

In the middle three quintile bands of wards, the discrepancy between observed mortality and that predicted in the light of class structure is not very large, varying between 3 and 13 per cent. However, at either end of the spectrum the discrepancy is much wider, with SMRs 31 per cent above and 40 per cent below predicted levels in the two extreme 10 per cent blocs. This means that the proportion and number of deaths which cannot be accounted for in terms of occupational class are greatest where mortality is highest, and decreases as we move from those areas with worst health to those with less bad health. In the worst 10 per cent band, nearly one-quarter of deaths (23 per cent of all deaths) may be regarded as 'excess' deaths, in the sense that they are unexplained by class composition; but this fraction falls sharply as overall mortality itself declines. Indeed, in more than half the wards of the Region there are fewer deaths than would be expected on the basis of class composition, and this pattern is most pronounced in the wards where mortality is lowest.

Figure 7.1: Standardising mortality for occupational Class across the Northern Region: actual and predicted patterns compared, 1981–3 (678 wards ranked according to mortality and divided into 10 per cent and 20 per cent bands)

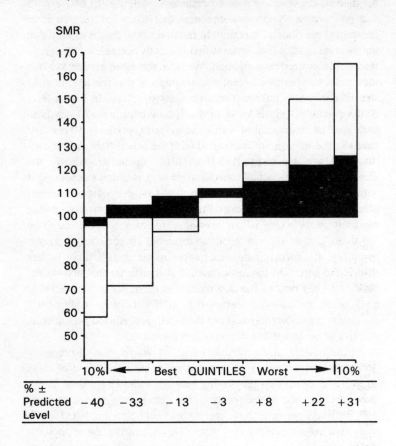

| % ±
Predicted
Level | − 40 | − 33 | − 13 | − 3 | + 8 | + 22 | + 31 |

Note: Actual SMRs for each quintile and extreme decile bands are represented by unshaded area. Predicted SMRs on basis of occupational class composition are represented by the shaded area. For calculation of predicted SMRs see note to Table 7.4.

The overall picture to emerge is clear and unambiguous, therefore, although it must be remembered that the predicted mortality figures take account of the class composition alone in the wards in each bloc and not the age distribution also. Despite this limitation, there is no evidence to suggest that at the two ends of the health spectrum the discrepancy between predicted and observed mortality would be greatly modified if it were possible to standardise for age and class simultaneously, even though that would be the most desirable procedure. We are confident, then, that the pattern reproduced in Figure 7.1 is broadly reliable.

The technique can be applied valuably to certain districts and counties, and in particular to groups of wards in Cleveland and Tyne and Wear, the two essentially urban counties of the Region, and those in which ward populations are larger than elsewhere. In Table 7.4 observed SMRs and SMRs predicted on the basis of class composition are contrasted in the 25 per cent of wards in each district where premature mortality is highest (see Table 4.2). It will

Table 7.4: Standardising mortality for Occupational Class in the 25 per cent of wards with highest mortality in each district in Cleveland and Tyne and Wear, 1981–83: actual and predicted patterns compared

District	All persons 0–64 SMR	SMR predicted on basis of class composition	% difference from prediction
Hartlepool	165	127	+ 30
Langbaurgh	167	138	+ 21
Middlesbrough	170	143	+ 19
Stockton	155	130	+ 19
Gateshead	160	128	+ 25
Newcastle	155	120	+ 29
North Tyneside	144	109	+ 32
South Tyneside	138	117	+ 18
Sunderland	136	128	+ 6

Note: The SMR predicted on the basis of class composition here has been derived from data on male deaths between 15 and 64, utilising occupational class death rates of England and Wales. The necessary assumption is made that a ward's overall class composition between 0 and 64 is identical to the male 15–64 composition. The formula is as follows (see also Appendix 3):

Male 15–64 expected deaths (applying England and Wales occupational class death rates)	÷	Male 15–64 expected deaths (applying England and Wales age-specific death rates)	× 100

be apparent that in every case, observed mortality is higher than that predicted, thus reflecting in a more localised form the evidence considered in Figure 7.1. Moreover, the wards in question in Middlesbrough and Langbaurgh not only experience the highest age-standardised mortality among the districts considered; they also have the highest predicted mortality. What this table also brings out, however, is the contrast between one district, Sunderland, where almost all the mortality in its worst wards is explicable in terms of class composition (observed mortality is only 6 per cent higher than that predicted); and four districts — North Tyneside, Hartlepool, Newcastle and Gateshead — where class composition alone still leaves a significant amount of the high mortality unexplained (observed mortality being between one-quarter and one-third higher than that predicted). It is these latter districts in which it appears to be the case that even after occupational class has been taken into account, large numbers of 'excess' deaths remain to be explained.

To conclude this chapter, we have shown that standardising for occupational class helps to explain some of the high mortality in areas of the North, given the proviso that it has not been possible to standardise for age and class together. Occupational class is clearly of major importance in explaining inequalities in health; but just as clearly, there is a need to go beyond occupational class (at least as it is presently defined) in explaining these inequalities. Broadly speaking, either there are factors independent of occupational class which contribute in substantial measure to any further explanation of excess deaths, or occupational class includes systematic variations in the experience of material deprivation which need to be revealed if a further large number of the observed excess deaths are to be explained. As will become clear in the next chapter, by taking into account the experience of deprivation, rather than occupational class alone, it is indeed possible to explain a larger part of the variations in mortality which occur.

8

Material Deprivation and the Explanation of Health Inequalities

Material deprivation turns out to be at least as valuable in explaining inequalities of health as occupational class. Having considered the distribution of ill-health (Chapter 4) and the prevalence of material deprivation (Chapter 5), the connection will now be examined more closely. For the Northern Region this chapter illustrates the analysis offered by the Working Group chaired by Sir Douglas Black, in which 'material deprivation' was broadly identified as the prime cause of inequalities in health (Black Report, 1980, pp. 193–5).

8.1 THE STRENGTH OF THE ASSOCIATION BETWEEN HEALTH AND DEPRIVATION

Previous chapters have described the close links between material conditions of life and health. We begin this chapter by presenting some of the key statistical correlations between the primary indicators used in this study. The inter-relationship between the deprivation variables is stronger than that between the health variables.

The relationships between the health and deprivation variables are shown in Table 8.1, in which the Overall Health Index and Overall Deprivation Index are also included. The table shows that, of the three separate health measures, permanent sickness is most strongly associated with each of the deprivation indicators; low birthweight has the weakest relationship with each of the deprivation indicators, though statistically, the correlation coefficients are still highly significant. Of the deprivation indicators the two which are most strongly associated with each of the health indicators are unemployment and the proportion of households which do not possess a car — the income surrogate. (Correlations among the sets of health and

107

Table 8.1: The relationship between the health and deprivation indicators for the Northern Region: Spearman rank correlation coefficients (678 wards)

Deprivation indicators	Persons 0–64 SMR	% Residents aged 16 and over permanently sick	% Live births under 2,800 gm	Overall Health Index
		Health Indicators		
% Unemployed	0.61	0.77	0.47	0.78
% Households with more persons than rooms	0.55	0.72	0.42	0.70
% Households with no car	0.61	0.80	0.47	0.80
% Households not owner-occupied	0.39	0.63	0.33	0.57
% Households with head in Class IIIM, IV or V	0.57	0.72	0.43	0.73
Overall Deprivation Index	0.62	0.84	0.48	0.82

Note: Spearman rank correlation coefficients, rather than Pearson product-moment correlation coefficients, have been calculated because the assumption for each pair of variables that the scores are from a bivariate normal population does not hold in every case. All of the above correlation coefficients are highly statistically significant of a strong association.

Figure 8.1: The relationship between health and deprivation in the Northern Region

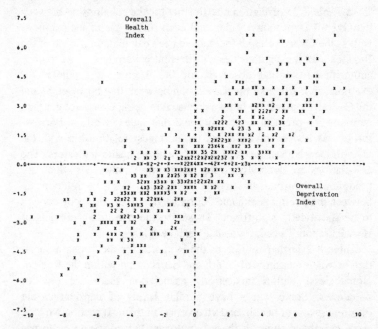

Note: Each 'X' represents one of the 678 wards; a number instead of an X indicates that more than one ward is situated at that point.

deprivation indicators are to be found in Appendix 5, Table A5.6.) In Table 8.1 all of the correlation coefficients are highly statistically significant of a strong association between each pair of variables. It is interesting to note that the correlation coefficients are generally highest for those relationships in which one member of the pair is an Overall Health or Deprivation Index. This adds to the arguments presented earlier for the operational representation of different elements of meaning in examining the distribution of the two phenomena, and drawing lessons for policy. One of the strongest relationships is that between the Overall Health Index and the Overall Deprivation Index: the correlation coefficient is 0.82 and the relationship is illustrated in a plot in Figure 8.1. By measuring the health of a ward in terms of three key dimensions (premature mortality, chronic sickness and disablement, and delayed development) and by incorporating different, and in some respects

109

complementary, measures of deprivation, the strong association between ill-health and deprivation can be demonstrated.

In Table 8.2 correlation coefficients for the relationship between the Overall Deprivation Index and each of the health indicators as well as the Overall Health Index have been calculated for each of the Regions's 29 local authorities. A different pattern emerges for some authorities from that observed for the Region as a whole: for example, in Hartlepool the association between low birthweight and the Overall Deprivation Index is unusual in being even stronger than that between premature mortality and that Index; while in Barrow-in-Furness low birthweight has the strongest relationship with the Overall Deprivation Index of any of the three health indicators. The associations are generally strongest for those authorities which are predominantly urban, and in only three authorities is the relationship between the overall health and deprivation indices not strong enough to be statistically significant. These are the non-urban districts of Berwick-upon-Tweed, Tynedale and Teesdale.

Table 8.2 further reinforces the evidence for the strong association between measures of health and deprivation within the Region. Nonetheless, within this strong association there are obvious paradoxes. Some wards have similar levels of deprivation but different levels of health, and vice versa. In the next section we look more closely at some of these paradoxes; before we go on to use regression analyses to consider, firstly, the relationship between ill-health and deprivation (section 8.3), and, secondly, the explanation for mortality differences in Tyne and Wear and Cleveland specifically (section 8.4).

8.2 PREDICTABLE AND PARADOXICAL PATTERNS OF HEALTH

As demonstrated above, there are extremely strong associations between overall health, overall deprivation and occupational class in the Northern Region, confirming a pattern which is well established (see, for example, the Black Report, 1980). However, the approach adopted in this study enables us to go beyond the demonstration of this connection, to identify some of its strengths and ambiguities. Inevitably there are variations in the extent to which local patterns reflect the general direction of evidence, with either more or less pronounced patterns of ill-health accompanying broadly similar levels of deprivation.

Certain paradoxes are evident from the overall regional pattern or when districts are compared. Thus, for example, the very strong correlation between low birthweight and overall deprivation in North Tyneside and Hartlepool may be set alongside the less strong association between these two indicators in the region as a whole, or the much weaker and scarcely significant correlation between the two in South Tyneside and Easington (Table 8.2). This discrepancy is puzzling, and raises the question as to why it is that the link between low birthweight and deprivation can be so evident in one district and yet so much less evident in a neighbouring district. There are, in addition, several local paradoxes: for example, wards with high female but low male mortality, or high mortality but good health on other criteria; or again considerable deprivation but rather better health than might have been anticipated. These illustrations are a reminder that the scientific explanation of social patterns of health is still in its early stages. The explanation of many such cases may require local knowledge and more detailed investigation than is possible where the canvas is as large as it is in this study. However, in this section we draw attention to some of the more striking anomalies and unexpected patterns of health.

While Figure 8.1 confirms the strong association between health and material circumstances, a look at the distribution of wards reveals that at any particular level of deprivation, wards are to be found which experience relatively better or worse health. This is of course inevitable, and serves as a reminder against too deterministic an interpretation of the link between the two. However, it is worth examining the spread of health experienced in wards with similar levels of deprivation in order to pick out any regularities there may be — any tendency for wards in some areas to have consistently worse health, and in other areas consistently better health, for a given level of deprivation.

To accomplish this we have looked first at the 34 wards which make up the most deprived 5 per cent of all wards in the region. These we have divided into two, distinguishing the half (17) with the worse and the half with the better overall health. We have then repeated the exercise for the next most deprived 5 per cent of wards. This simple method does indeed reveal in this case quite definite regularities. Among the most deprived wards of all are five in Sunderland, each in the group with less bad overall health, and eight wards on the south side of the Tees, six of which are in the group with worse health. Similarly, among the next most deprived wards are six South Tyneside wards, all in the group with less bad health,

111

Table 8.2: The relationship between Overall Deprivation and each of the health indicators in the 29 local authorities of the Northern Region: Spearman rank correlation coefficients

Local authority	Spearman rank correlation coefficients				Number of Wards	Value for Significance[a]
	Overall deprivation versus					
	Persons 0–64 SMR	Permanent sickness	Low birthweight	Overall health		
Northern Region	0.62	0.84	0.48	0.82	678	0.10
Hartlepool	0.71	0.93	0.76	0.84	17	0.50
Langbaurgh	0.74	0.84	0.59	0.84	26	0.40
Middlesbrough	0.79	0.93	0.70	0.93	25	0.41
Stockton	0.58	0.92	0.52	0.83	30	0.37
Allerdale	0.32	0.76	0.21	0.57	34	0.35
Barrow-in-Furness	0.46	0.43	0.76	0.81	13	0.59
Carlisle	0.52	0.75	0.50	0.78	23	0.43
Copeland	0.77	0.70	0.35	0.81	26	0.40
Eden	0.25	0.53	0.36	0.48	28	0.38
South Lakeland	0.34	0.45	0.18	0.42	47	0.29
Chester-le-Street	0.45	0.90	0.30	0.79	17	0.50
Darlington	0.73	0.89	0.65	0.87	25	0.41
Derwentside	0.28	0.69	0.38	0.73	23	0.43
Durham	0.51	0.91	0.60	0.84	24	0.42
Easington	0.41	0.53	0.41	0.56	26	0.40
Sedgefield	0.25	0.49	0.57	0.54	22	0.44
Teesdale	0.18	0.35	0.12	0.19	19	0.47
Wear Valley	0.54	0.92	0.47	0.81	21	0.45

Alnwick	0.60	0.34	0.55	0.61	17	0.50
Berwick	0.31	0.55	0.07	0.46	16	0.52
Blyth Valley	0.70	0.82	0.63	0.85	17	0.50
Castle Morpeth	0.37	0.67	0.33	0.76	21	0.45
Tynedale	0.28	0.46	0.06	0.30	32	0.36
Wansbeck	0.81	0.82	0.01	0.75	16	0.52
Gateshead	0.78	0.69	0.62	0.85	22	0.44
Newcastle	0.85	0.93	0.73	0.94	26	0.40
North Tyneside	0.85	0.93	0.85	0.93	20	0.46
South Tyneside	0.50	0.72	0.48	0.79	20	0.46
Sunderland	0.79	0.73	0.38	0.86	25	0.41

Note: [a] Value above which correlation coefficient is statistically significant at 5% (two-tailed test)

whereas three out of the four Middlesbrough wards are in the group with worse health. In all, there are 14 Sunderland and South Tyneside wards in these two groups, none of which is among those with worse health. By contrast, there are twelve Middlesbrough and Langbaurgh wards featured, nine of which are among those with worse health.

Among the most deprived wards of all, the 17 with worse overall health owe their position primarily to high premature mortality, with low birthweight a secondary factor and permanent sickness of least importance. In the wards characterised by slightly less severe deprivation, all three health criteria are important in accounting for the difference in overall health, with low birthweight being a more pronounced factor than the still considerable disparities in mortality and morbidity.

If the marked contrast in mortality and low birthweight between Sunderland or South Tyneside and the south side of the Tees provides one apparent paradox, the contrast between Sunderland and parts of Newcastle, Gateshead and North Tyneside provides another — for the five Sunderland wards of Town End Farm, South Hylton, Southwick, Thorney Close and Castletown represent the most striking group of extremely deprived wards in a single district in Tyne and Wear. Yet these areas experience distinctly better health than wards of equivalent or ostensibly lower levels of deprivation in these other three Tyne and Wear districts, Gateshead providing the sharpest contrast here.

Within Newcastle itself there seems to be a distinction between the east and west sides of the city, with a tendency towards generally worse health among the deprived wards of the west than among the deprived wards of the east. West City and Scotswood in the west, and Walker in the east, epitomise this contrast. The indicators of deprivation provide few clues towards an explanation: yet even if the explanation were to be pursued in the different kinds of historical development shaping east and west Newcastle — for example, in housing patterns, population stability, male and female employment traditions — some puzzling discrepancies between the health experience of seemingly similar areas would remain. The comparison between the two shipyard-dominated wards of Walker and Howdon (North Tyneside) is a case in point. On almost every criterion Walker is slightly but definitely more deprived than Howdon, yet it is Howdon which has quite unambiguously the worse health record at the present time, on all three of our main health indicators, as well as on a supplementary criterion such as the SMR for the 65–74 age band. The picture becomes still more surprising when male and female mortality patterns are differentiated. Walker actually has the higher male premature mortality (SMR of 157 compared with 136 in Howdon), but it has extremely low female mortality whereas Howdon's is particularly high (SMRs of 78 and 170). Great caution is needed when interpreting findings such as these which are based on the comparison between single wards. Nevertheless, there does appear to be a paradox here which the data enable us to identify, but not to explain.

Turning now to Durham, it is noteworthy that only nine wards figure among the 68 most deprived, with just two each from Easington and Wear Valley, the districts in which ill-health is most pronounced in the county. We have found that the measures of deprivation used in this study generally correlate more strongly with health indices in urban rather than non-urban areas, and especially strongly in the conurbations of Tyne and Wear and Cleveland. Whether this is in part a product of larger ward sizes in the conurbations, and the greater possibility of freakish or unrepresentative health patterns emerging in the smaller wards of Durham, Cumbria and Northumberland; or whether the measures of deprivation adopted here do less justice to the realities of deprivation in non-urban areas than in the cities is a moot point, and difficult to ascertain within the confines of the census data. We return to it in the next section.

What can be said with regard to Durham is that the old county planning designation of rural communities by the letters A, B, C or D provides a significant guide to current health patterns in many parts of the county, but nowhere more so than in Easington (Durham County Council, 1954, 1969, which abolished the letters whilst retaining the substance of the designation). Category D communities were the dying villages which it was not official policy to resurrect, and since the 1950s most of these have virtually disappeared from the map. Today, the communities most likely to be in need of services and infrastructural improvement are those which were formerly classified as Category C settlements; and in Easington, for instance, the list of ex-category C villages offers a ready clue to the areas of bad health in the majority of cases: Wheatley Hill, Wingate, Shotton, Station Town, Thornley, Horden, and Easington Colliery and Village, are all examples. The now defunct classification is indicative of a form of deprivation in itself, as certain localities were made relatively marginal in terms of development plans. What this study shows is that in many of these areas ill-health goes hand-in-hand with such social and economic marginality. Moreover, it should be clear that it would be misleading to put down Durham's pattern of ill-health to the costs of coal mining alone, when it is borne in mind that in east Durham and Easington it is female, not male, premature mortality which is so great.

In this section we have qualified the overall picture of an extremely strong association between health and deprivation by drawing attention to some of the main complexities and paradoxes which emerge from a close examination of the findings. The instances we have looked at are not anomalies to the extent that they actually run counter to the overall association between ill-health and deprivation. There scarcely exist any affluent wards in the region with bad health, any more than there are to be found highly deprived wards with good health. Thus, for example, among the most affluent 20 per cent of wards in the region (as ranked on the overall deprivation index), there are none to be found among the 20 per cent with the poorest health overall, and only four among the 40 per cent with the poorest health. Conversely, and mirroring this pattern, among the most deprived 20 per cent of wards in the region, not one has health good enough to rank among the best 20 per cent (on the overall health index), and only two have health good enough to rank them among the best 40 per cent. Affluence is generally associated with good health; and pronounced deprivation almost invariably means poor health.

However, where the paradoxes do arise is in the matter of just how bad this poor health may be. South Tyneside's and Sunderland's poor health is not the same as Middlesbrough's or Newcastle's or Gateshead's at the present time, for example. Moreover, this is particularly notable in view of the fact that at least until the early 1970s mortality was especially high in many areas on the south bank of the Tyne. It is to the further statistical analysis of some of these variations that we now turn.

8.3 EXPLAINING INEQUALITIES IN HEALTH: REGRESSION ANALYSIS

A major objective of this study has been to seek explanations for the observed inequalities in health between different wards. This theme is continued in this section, in which regression techniques are used to analyse the data. In a regression the dependent variable and one or more independent variables are analysed together, in order to determine how much of the variance in the dependent variable can be 'explained' by a combination of one or more of the independent variables. In this context the Overall Health Index is the dependent variable and the deprivation and class variables are the independent variables: the analysis seeks to explain the variance, or inequality, in overall health in terms of certain measures of deprivation and class. The data are analysed for the Northern Region as a whole and also separately for each of the five counties.

In the region as a whole, overall health is most strongly associated with the car ownership variable — the proxy for low income — and unemployment, important though the two housing variables are. This regional pattern is found to be repeated at county level, for car ownership and unemployment emerge as the two most consistently important variables for each of the five counties (see Appendix 5, Table A5.7). There are, nevertheless, differences between counties in the strength of each of the deprivation variables, with the strongest associations found in Cleveland and Tyne and Wear — the two almost entirely urban counties — with Durham following on all variables except one.

The next stage is to carry out stepwise regressions of the Overall Health Index on just the four main deprivation variables. This will take further the examination of the differences between counties. In a stepwise regression the independent variables (here the deprivation variables) enter the regression equation one by one, depending on the contribution which each makes to reducing that variance in the dependent variable (here the Overall Health Index) which is so far unexplained. Thus, if an independent variable does not make a significant ($p < .05$ here) contribution to reducing the unexplained variance, then it does not enter the regression, even though it may be strongly correlated with the dependent variable.

The regression results for the Region and for each of the five counties are summarised in Table 8.3. For each regression the deprivation variables are listed in the order in which they entered the regression equation — that is, in order of decreasing contribution to the variance of the Overall Health Index. Thus in all of the six regressions the first variable to enter was either the car ownership variable or the unemployment variable. The regression on all 678 wards shows that each of the four components of the Overall Deprivation Index make a significant contribution to explaining the variation in overall health within the Region. It is worth remembering at this point that the choice of these four components was based firstly on the decision to distinguish between predominantly material and predominantly social aspects of deprivation, and then to choose four relatively broad indicators of material deprivation which are available from census data and which could be demonstrated to bear differing relationships

117

Table 8.3: Regressions of Overall Health Index separately on deprivation and class indicators for each Northern Region county: proportion of variance in overall health explained by each regression

County	Combination of some or all of the four main deprivation indicators chosen by stepwise regression	Percentage of households with head in manual class	Percentage of households with head in Class IV or V
Region	% Households with no car % Unemployed % Households overcrowded % Households not owner occupied } 65%	48	32
Tyne and Wear	% Households with no car % Households overcrowded % Households not owner occupied } 78%	60	76
Cleveland	% Unemployed % Households with no car } 81%	60	64
Cumbria	% Unemployed % Households with no car % Households overcrowded } 49%	33	27
Durham	% Households with no car % Households not owner occupied % Households overcrowded } 56%	49	34
Northumberland	% Households with no car % Households overcrowded } 52%	33	3

For example, across the region as a whole (i.e. 678 wards) it is possible to explain 65% of the variance in overall health by a combination of the four main deprivation indicators, whereas only 48% and 32% respectively can be explained by the two class variables.

to material living standards — access to earnings and the facilities of employment; space in the home; security and wealth; and (in the case of owning a car) current income. It is some vindication of the original decision to discover that all four components do play a significant part in explaining the distribution of health across the region, with car ownership having the strongest explanatory value, and housing tenure the weakest of the four.

However, when the individual counties are compared different patterns emerge. In Cleveland and Tyne and Wear the relationship between overall health and deprivation is particularly strong (the percentages of variance explained are 81 and 78 respectively), but the emphasis of the different components of deprivation is quite different. Unemployment is the most important variable in the Cleveland result, but it does not appear at all in that for Tyne and Wear. The only variable to appear in the results for both counties is that for car ownership. It is interesting to note that this is the only one of the four variables to appear in the regressions for all five counties. Overcrowding features in the case of four out of five counties, though nowhere as the main variable; and housing tenure (the percentage of households not owner occupied) features only in Tyne and Wear and Durham.

While in the two essentially urban counties the deprivation indicators combine to explain around 80 per cent of the variance in overall health, in Durham this falls to 56 per cent and in Cumbria and Northumberland still lower, even though these values are still statistically highly significant. These findings raise an important question: Is health less closely related to material conditions in rural than in urban areas? Or do our deprivation indicators most accurately reflect and identify urban rather than rural deprivation? Positive answers to both provide possible interpretations, but perhaps the determining factor is the smaller ward size in parts of Durham, and throughout Cumbria and Northumberland.

The previous chapter described the use of occupational class as an explanatory variable (mainly in the context of premature mortality), and it is natural at this point to introduce occupational class variables into the regression analysis, and to ask whether they explain more of the variance in overall health than has already been explained by the use of deprivation variables. Regressions have been run on the Overall Health Index firstly on the manual class variable and then on the Class IV and V variable, and the results are summarised in Table 8.3. Across the Region as a whole, 48 per cent of the variance in overall health can be explained by the manual class variable and

119

32 per cent by the Class IV and V variable. Thus, neither of the class variables is as effective an explanatory tool as the combination of the four deprivation variables, which explain as much as 65 per cent of the variance in overall health across the Region.

As before, when the individual counties are compared, different patterns emerge. In Tyne and Wear the Class IV and V variable explains almost as much of the variance as is explained by the three selected deprivation variables (76 per cent and 78 per cent respectively). Only in Tyne and Wear and Cleveland does the percentage of households in Class IV and V explain more than the percentage in all the manual classes, but in Cleveland the difference is only 4 per cent. In the other three counties it is the percentage in all the manual classes which explains more than the percentage in Class IV and V, the greatest difference being in Northumberland where 33 per cent of the variance is explained by the former but only 3 per cent by the latter. However, it should be emphasised that in each county it is the combined effect of the deprivation variables which explains the greater proportion of the variance in overall health.

We also considered the possibility that by enlarging the set of deprivation variables at our disposal, and including either one of the two class variables just mentioned, we might be able to explain a significantly greater proportion of the variance in health. The results are summarised in Appendix 5, Table A5.8, and they indicate that by enlarging the range of independent variables, almost no extra explanatory power is gained. In the Region as a whole there is merely a 1 per cent improvement, and the same applies in every county except Durham, where there is a 5 per cent improvement. What is more, with the exception of Tyne and Wear, where the Class IV and V variable is the leading one, in all the other results the leading variable remains car ownership or unemployment. The importance of the car ownership indicator cannot be stressed too strongly: it appears in every regression. This exercise would appear to offer strong confirmation of the approach taken in this study towards the choice of indicators of deprivation, substantiating our argument that, providing different aspects of material living standards are covered, a small range of indicators can provide reliable representation of geographical variation.

We have shown in this section that the use of indicators of deprivation helps to account for a greater part of health inequalities than the use of occupational class. This is as true in Cleveland and Tyne and Wear, where occupational class nevertheless has considerable explanatory value, as in Cumbria and Northumberland, where class provides a much more wayward guide to health patterns at ward level. Over the Region as a whole, the improvement in explanatory value achieved with deprivation indicators, by comparison with class indicators, is impressive. At the same time, within the strong, region-wide association between ill-health and deprivation, it appears that different aspects of deprivation take on greater or lesser prominence in different parts of the region.

8.4 EXPLAINING MORTALITY IN CLEVELAND AND TYNE AND WEAR: REGRESSION ANALYSIS

In this section we return to an observation which has often recurred throughout this study: the different mortality levels experienced in the most adversely affected wards of Cleveland and Tyne and Wear. This difference is best exemplified by the contrast between the south Teesside area, on the one hand, and South Tyneside and Sunderland on the other. We shall employ the regression technique to examine how much the generally higher mortality in Cleveland may be explained statistically in terms of its deprivation, and indeed, whether or not there remain excess deaths, even after the prevalence of depriva-tion has been taken into account, in each of the districts within these two counties. For this purpose, the 98 Cleveland wards and the 113 Tyne and Wear wards have been grouped together. As a first step, selected correlation coefficients have been calculated. These are given in Table 8.4, and once again confirm the strong association between premature mortality and each of the four main deprivation indices, although it will be seen that the owner-occupation variable is not as strongly correlated with mortality as the other three. In addition, when a regression is run of the premature mortality indicator on all four deprivation variables simultaneously, as much as 63 per cent of the variance in mortality in these two counties is explained.

The regression equation resulting has been applied to the 211 wards to produce a predicted SMR value for the deaths of all people under 65, which has then been compared with the observed value. This exer-cise is the logical counterpart of the comparison in the previous chapter of mortality predicted on the basis of occupational class with that actually occurring. However, there is one important difference: in standardising for occupational class, national class mortality patterns were taken as the yardstick against which to evaluate the variations occurring in the North. However, in standardising for the impact of deprivation, predicted SMRs have been produced on the basis of

Table 8.4: The relationship between premature mortality and the deprivation indicators in Cleveland and Tyne and Wear combined: correlation coefficients

	Persons 0–64 SMR
% unemployed	0.78
% households with no car	0.69
% households with more persons than rooms	0.71
% households not owner-occupied	0.56

Note: Cleveland and Tyne and Wear together comprise 211 wards.

deprivation solely within the two counties under consideration. In other words, we have attempted to account for local mortality variations not by reference to national levels of deprivation but specifically by reference to the relevant sub-regional levels. This inevitably enhances the 'fit' between predicted and observed mortality, because it is the procedure which enables prediction to come as close as possible to the level of mortality actually occurring. Even so, as will be seen, a number of discrepancies remain.

The findings are presented in Tables 8.5 and 8.6. In Table 8.5, observed and predicted SMRs are set alongside each other, not only for the one-quarter of wards with the highest mortality in each district (as in Table 7.4), but also in the quarter of wards with the lowest mortality. A fairly consistent pattern is apparent, if the two extremes of the health spectrum are compared. All of the bands of wards with high mortality except one experience higher death rates than might be expected from a knowledge of their level of deprivation; whereas all of the bands of wards with low mortality experience lower death rates than might be expected. These data provide confirmation of the pattern illustrated in Figure 7.1. At the low mortality end of the scale, it is interesting to note that only in three of the districts is affluence great enough to produce the expectaion of mortality at below the national average (i.e. 100), and even in these cases the predicted values are scarcely below 100. Moreover, in South Tyneside the gap between predicted mortality levels in the highest and lowest 25 per cent bands is very small, evidence of the considerable socio-economic homogeneity of that district, and the even spread of measured deprivation.

What stands out in three of Cleveland's four districts — Hartlepool, Langbaurgh and above all Middlesbrough — is that in the worst quarter of wards mortality predicted on the basis of deprivation is higher than anywhere in Tyne and Wear. In particular, the

Table 8.5: Assessing mortality in the light of deprivation in Cleveland and Tyne and Wear

District	Quarter of wards with highest mortality			Quarter of wards with lowest mortality		
	0–64 SMR (persons)	SMR predicted on basis of deprivation	% ± difference from prediction	0–64 SMR (persons)	SMR predicted on basis of deprivation	% ± difference from prediction
Hartlepool	165	148	+ 11	87	110	− 21
Langbaurgh	167	148	+ 12	82	102	− 20
Middlesbrough	170	163	+ 4	86	96	− 10
Stockton	155	137	+ 14	86	99	− 14
Gateshead	160	137	+ 17	99	102	− 3
Newcastle	155	142	+ 9	93	104	− 11
North Tyneside	144	132	+ 9	81	99	− 18
South Tyneside	138	132	+ 4	101	114	− 12
Sunderland	136	142	− 4	96	106	− 9

Note: The SMR predicted on the basis of deprivation is given by the regression equation ($R^2 = 0.63$):

Predicted SMR = 66.4718 + (2.1493 × % unemployed)
+ (0.3582 × % households with no car)
+ (1.6108 × % households overcrowded)
− (0.1179 × % households not owner occupied)

very high mortality occurring in Middlesbrough, to which we have repeatedly drawn attention, appears to be almost entirely accounted for by the deprivation prevalent in the wards concerned, with the level of mortality predicted being just 4 per cent below that observed. In Hartlepool and Langbaurgh, on the other hand, as also in Stockton, there remain small but nevertheless significant proportions of deaths which are excessive in the light of known levels of deprivation. In these worst-hit wards, actual and predicted mortality levels are closest in Middlesbrough, South Tyneside and Sunderland, although the last of these stands out as the sole district where expected mortality is higher than actual mortality. In Newcastle and North Tyneside, deprivation explains far more of the high mortality than was achieved by taking account of occupational class (compare, for example, Table 7.4). Only in Gateshead does a notable proportion of the high mortality remain unexplained by deprivation, the figures here representing just a small improvement on those obtained by standardising for class. In this connection, Bede and Deckham wards stand out as experiencing far greater numbers of deaths than would be predicted on the basis of their deprivation, considerable though that deprivation is.

Table 8.6 extends this discussion of wards with high mortality by taking three clusters of adjacent wards, which between them account for the most significant large blocs of severe deprivation in Cleveland and Tyne and Wear. Two of these clusters — covering the south bank of the Tees from Thornaby to the coast, and straddling the Tyne in Newcastle and Gateshead — have already been examined in Chapter 4; the third[6] covers the north and west of Sunderland on both sides of the Wear. The table contrasts the mortality predicted on the basis of both occupational class and deprivation in the three blocs of wards, but chiefly it highlights the way in which areas with ostensibly similar class composition and, more importantly, similar levels of deprivation, nevertheless diverge to a significant degree in their mortality patterns. It is true that the Teesside bloc is confirmed as being slightly but demonstrably more deprived than the other two, on the basis of its predicted SMR. The greatest contrast is arguably between the Tyneside and Wearside wards, which are so closely comparable on the criterion of deprivation, yet experience strikingly different mortality. There can be no disputing the fact that death rates in these deprived Sunderland wards are high, in national terms; but the point to bring out is that they are actually by some margin lower than might be predicted from knowledge of their deprivation, reinforcing an observation made at various points in this study. Moreover, they

Table 8.6: Comparison of mortality taking account of Occupational Class and deprivation in three ward clusters

Name of cluster	Total population	0–64 SMR (persons)	SMR predicted on basis of class composition	% ± difference from prediction	SMR predicted on basis of deprivation	% ± difference from prediction
1 South Tees	86,000	164	134	+ 22	156	+ 5
2 Central Tyneside	54,000	170	130	+ 31	145	+ 18
3 North and West Sunderland	80,000	130	125	+ 4	144	– 10

Note: The SMR predicted on the basis of deprivation is given by the regression equation ($R^2 = 0.63$):

Predicted SMR = 66.4718 + (2.1493 × % unemployed)
    + (0.3582 × % households with no car)
    + (1.6108 × % households overcrowded)
    – (0.1179 × % households not owner occupied)

represent a very different health experience from that in the heart of Newcastle and Gateshead, where death rates are distinctly higher than expected rates, leaving a significant proportion of excess deaths which cannot be explained.

Contrasting with both of these examples, the band of wards on the south side of the Tees reveals a pattern of high mortality which appears to be largely explained by an overall level of deprivation which is unmatched — in terms of severity and the size of the population affected — in the entire Region. The sheer scale of poverty and economic depression in these wards has its counterpart in the very high mortality which is likewise unmatched elsewhere in the Region for its consistency across such a large population. However, if the overall pattern of high mortality across these 15 wards appears to be largely accounted for by the severity of the deprivation experienced there, there is nevertheless within this bloc one area immediately to the east of Middlesbrough, comprising the wards of South Bank, Grangetown and Church Lane, where extremely high observed mortality (reflected in the SMR of 186) is 12 per cent higher than predicted on the basis of admittedly extreme deprivation. This suggests that it may be unwise to rule out the impact of additional factors in some areas of south Teesside, just as it would be in the bloc of wards examined in the centre of Tyneside.

There are at least two possibilities. The first has to do with the census indicators themselves, and their capacity to reflect social reality. At best they do of course provide only a rough guide to a complex social picture; but more than that, the suspicion exists that in places where deprivation is very severe, census indices may be inadequate for the task of registering the effects of the many factors which compound one another. In other words, the cumulative impact of severe deprivation may be more acute than the sum of its separate parts — and certainly more than those parts which are measureable by means of census or similar indicators. In the South Bank area, therefore, as also in the central part of Newcastle and Gateshead, the reality of deprivation may have been underestimated.

A second possibility also needs to be taken into account, however, one which is particularly relevant to Teesside. This also has a bearing on the criteria of deprivation deployed in this study. The indicators we have chosen reflect, in our judgement, necessary dimensions of the experience of deprivation, but these are by no means sufficient dimenions, on account of the limitations of available data; and a comprehensive approach to material deprivation ought ideally to include an index of the environmental pollution, and specifically the air pollution, experienced in different areas. In Teesside, the possible consequences for health of air pollution emanating — especially in the not so distant past — from the massive chemical and steel complexes come on top of the severest deprivation, complicating attempts to disentangle the various factors. Yet the issue of air pollution is one which must be raised, given the unusually high mortality found in large parts of Teesside.

In Teesside today, air pollution levels, as monitored in smoke and sulphur dioxide emissions and deposits of undissolved solids, have improved dramatically since 1960: on these criteria, for instance, Middlesbrough now compares favourably with many towns and cities in the south of England. Several observations should be made, however. In looking at the factors underlying patterns of mortality, firstly, some of the determinants are to be found in past rather than present conditions. The impact of air pollution on health is in part a legacy of the worse conditions prevailing 15 years or more ago, and that legacy will be reflected in mortality rates well into the future. Secondly, even though there has been a great improvement in smoke and sulphur dioxide emissions and other forms of air pollution, and even though this improvement has benefited most those areas which were formerly the worst affected, the longstanding contrast between the more and less polluted areas nevertheless remains at the present time. The unequal experience of air pollution may fortunately be lessening, and not widening, but still persists to this day. The third observation to be made is that not all forms of air pollution are monitored with anything approaching the regularity and breadth of coverage of smoke, sulphur dioxide and undissolved solids. We cannot conclude that because in some respects air in Teesside compares favourably with the air in cities in southern England, it does so in every respect.

We conclude, then, with further questions rather than answers. The high mortality along the south bank of the Tees and in the heart of Tyneside owes much, we consider, to the severe poverty and deprivation experienced there (as measured by census indicators), but in both areas death rates are so very high that this explanation is not wholly satisfactory. By contrast, in Sunderland's most deprived wards death rates are not as high as might be anticipated, raising the question of how that state of affairs has been attained, and what factors have helped to counteract and modify the impact of deprivation on health. These are questions which require more detailed and intensive probing than we can undertake within the framework of the methodology used in this study.

9

The Widening Mortality Gap
in Britain and the North

During each decade the Registrar General publishes a new analysis of mortality which allows different industries and occupations to be compared, and progress in reducing the number of deaths to be calculated. These decennial supplements, as they are called, allow trends in inequalities between occupational groups and classes to be followed. The latest report was published in July 1986 (OPCS, 1986). Its most important evidence concerns the widening difference between occupational classes. In 1980 the Black Research Working Group had called specific attention to this trend, which had taken a number of forms (Black Report, 1980, especially Chapter 3). The phenomenon of widening inequality is confirmed by the latest evidence. This chapter will first describe and discuss that evidence and then go on to examine the manner in which the evidence is presented by the Registrar General. Secondly, the chapter will compare the North with the national pattern, on the basis of the official statistics of occupational mortality.

Table 9.1 sets out the trends for men in the relative mortality of different occupational classes. On the adjusted figures the SMR in the last 50 years of unskilled manual workers has increased from a figure 23 per cent higher than that of professional workers to a figure 77 per cent higher. The SMR of partly skilled workers has increased from a figure 9 per cent higher than that of managerial and administrative workers to a figure 53 per cent higher. While some doubts have been and are being expressed about the reliability of some of the data assigned to Class V of unskilled manual workers (see, in particular, OPCS, 1986, pp. 42–6), it has to be remembered that the widening trend in inequality applies generally among ranked occupational classes and especially to Class IV. In 1981 occupational Class IV accounted for 22.8 per cent and Class V 6.1 per cent

Table 9.1: Mortality of men by Occupational Class, over five decades (Standardised Mortality Ratios — England and Wales)

Period	Occupational Class					
	I Professional	II Managerial and administrative	III Non-manual	III Manual	IV Partly skilled manual	V Unskilled manual
1930–2	90	94	—	97	102	111
1949–53[a]	86	92	—	101	104	118
1959–63	76	81	—	100	103	143
adjusted[b]	(75)					(127)
1970–2	77	81	99	106	114	137
adjusted[b]	(75)					(121)
1979–80 and 1982–3	66	76	94	106	116	165
adjusted[c]	(70)					(124)

Source: For years prior to 1979–80 see the Black Report (1980). p. 65; and also OPCS (1978), p. 174. For 1979–83 see OPCS (1986).

Notes: a. Corrected figures as published in Registrar General's Decennial Supplement, England and Wales, 1961: Occupational Mortality Tables, London, HMSO, 1971, p. 22

b. Occupations in 1959–63 and 1970–72 have been re-classified according to the 1950 classification for purposes of adjusting the classes at the extremes, I and V. The Registrar General has given higher adjusted SMR figures for class V than given here, ie 134 and 123 respectively for 1959–63 and 1970–72 (OPCS, 1978 p. 174)

c. The adjusted figure of 70 for class I is given by OPCS after allowing for occupational re-classification between 1970 and 1980. "Changes in the other classes due to the new classification are minimal" (OPCS (1986) p. 45.) The adjusted figure of 124 for class V, also quoted by OPCS, really applies to the longer (and earlier) period 1971–81 and is drawn from the Longitudinal Survey. Further secondary analysis of the data is unlikely to produce a lower "adjusted" figure.

Table 9.2: Mortality of married and single women by Occupational Class over two decades (Standardised Mortality Ratios — England and Wales)

Period	Age-group	Occupational Class						
		I	II	III Non-manual	III Manual	IV	V	
Married								
1959–63	(15–64)	77	83	—	103	—	105	141
1970–2	(15–64)	82	87	92	115	119	135	
1979–80, 82–3	(20–59)	76	84	93	110	125	157	
Single								
1959–63	(15–64)	83	88	—	90	—	108	121
1970–2	(15–64)	110	79	92	108	114	138	
1979–80, 82–3	(20–59)	72	69	80	110	105	121	

Source: Registrar General's Decennial Supplement, 1961, pp. 91 and 503; OPCS, 1978, p. 211; and OPCS, 1986, p. 26.

of the classifiable male population, compared respectively with Class I at 6.0 per cent and Class II at 23.4 per cent (OPCS, 1986, Table GP2).

Table 9.2 gives corresponding information for married and single women for a shorter span of years. For married women, classified according to husband's occupation, the same trend can be seen as for men. Again, doubts about the data for occupational Class V have to be set against the pronounced and steady increase in the SMR for occupational Class IV. This class accounts for 22 per cent of the female population which can be classified, compared with only 7 per cent of the population in Class V. The figures in Table 9.2 need to be scrutinised with some care, not only because of the difficulty in classifying women by occupational class (OPCS, 1986, p. 24) but also because the age-group selected for primary analysis in the latest report differs from that for previous reports. The reservations apply in particular to the smaller numbers of deaths for single women, for which SMRs are given in the lower part of the table. The deaths of single women in the tables comprise only 10 per cent of women's deaths which are classified, and there were in the latest period covered (1979–80, 82–3) only 168 deaths in Class I and 401 in Class V. This may help to explain the unevenness of any trend in the data. The SMR of 121 is hard to interpret, since an SMR of 297 is given elsewhere (OPCS, 1986, p. 128) for the 233 deaths in Britain as a whole for Occupation Unit 160 (General Labourers).

Table 9.3: Mortality rates per 100,000 and as a percentage of rates for Occupational Classes I and II combined (1949–83, England and Wales, men and married women)

Sex	Age	Years	I and II	IV and V	IV and V as percentage of I and II
Males	25–34	1949–53	124	180	145
		1959–63	81	143	177
		1970–2	72	141	196
		1979–83	60	132	220
	35–44	1949–53	226	331	146
		1959–63	175	300	171
		1970–2	169	305	180
		1979–83	126	279	221
	45–54	1949–53	712	895	126
		1959–63	544	842	155
		1970–2	554	894	161
		1979–83	451	833	185
	55–64	1949–53	2097	2339	112
		1959–63	1804	2433	135
		1970–2	1710	2409	141
		1979–83	1405	2272	162
Females (married)	25–34	1949–53	85	141	166
		1959–63	51	77	151
		1970–2	42	68	162
		1979–83	34	58	170
	35–44	1949–53	170	226	133
		1959–63	123	186	151
		1970–2	118	193	164
		1979–83	92	153	166
	45–54	1949–53	427	513	120
		1959–63	323	455	141
		1970–2	337	510	151
		1979–83	279	475	170
	55–64	1949–53	1098	1226	112
		1959–63	818	1129	138
		1970–2	837	1131	135
		1979–83	(595)	(919)	(154)

Source: For the three periods 1949–53, 1959–63 and 1970–2; the Black Report, 1980, p. 68 (as derived from OPCS). For 1979–80 and 1982–3, OPCS, 1986, Microfiche Tables GP2, GP8, GD2, GD6.
Note: 1979–83 data for married women estimated.

Table 9.3 reproduces mortality rates from the last four decennial supplements and compares combined occupational Classes IV and V with I and II for selected adult age-groups. In each case substantial sections of the male and female populations are compared, thus ruling out the kind of reservations which might be attached to the interpretation of trends in mortality of small population categories. Thus, for 1979–83 the mortality rates of 29 per cent of males in the poorest classes (IV and V) are being compared with those of 27 per cent in the richest classes (I and II). The corresponding figures for married women are 29 per cent and 25 per cent.

For 10-year age-groups the trend for men aged 25–64 is regular, and unmistakeable. Relative to the poorer classes the mortality rates of the richer classes have substantially diminished since 1949. Of course, the 'absolute' mortality rates of combined occupational Classes IV and V have also diminished during three decades but not consistently and, at the older ages, only to a small extent. In 1979–83 the male mortality rate in England and Wales for those aged 45–54 was only 7 per cent lower, and for those aged 55–64 only 3 per cent lower, than in 1949–53. Even at these older ages the mortality rates of the two richest classes had diminished by 37 per cent and 33 per cent respectively. At younger ages the gain has been larger still. For men aged 25–34 mortality rates of occupational Classes I and II are less than half of what they were in 1949–53.

For women aged 25–34 there has been a similar trend since 1959 but if the figures for 1949–53, which show a larger differential than in the succeeding two decades, are added, then the change cannot be said to be consistent throughout the period. However, this is the only exception for the long span of years under consideration. The mortality rates for women in each 10-year age-group from 35 to 64, like those for men, have become more unequal, though a little less sharply. Again, among older women as among older men, the mortality rates of the poorer occupational classes have declined only by a small amount since 1949–53. For the 45–54 age-group, for example, the rates declined by only 7 per cent, whereas for the richer classes of that age, the rates declined by 35 per cent.

The change to which attention is called is not just one which applies to the categories at the extremes of the occupational class distribution. Table 9.4 shows for men that during the latest period for which information exists, the reduction of mortality was greatest in occupational Class I, and smaller in each succeeding class, with an increase attributed to occupational Class V. When deaths are grouped by cause and then analysed by class, another change becomes manifest. The class gradient observed for all deaths now applies to a larger number of different causes of death, and fewer causes are associated with an inverse class gradient.

In 1980 the Black Research Working Group pointed out that

Table 9.4: Trends in male mortality by Class 1970–83 (England and Wales): age-standardised deaths rates (per 1000)

Occupational Class	1970–2 (ages 15–64)	1979–80, and 1982–3 (ages 20–64)	Percentage improvement
I Professional	4.62	3.71	+ 20
II Senior administrative and managerial	4.86	4.18	+ 14
III Skilled non-manual	5.91	5.21	+ 12
III Skilled manual	6.33	5.79	+ 9
IV Partly skilled manual	6.81	6.41	+ 6
V Unskilled manual	8.32	9.09	− 9
All	5.97	5.43	+ 9

Source: OPCS, 1978, p. 37; and OPCS, 1986 Microfiche Table GD19.

deaths from some diseases which had previously been relatively more numerous in the richer than the poorer classes, or as numerous as in the poorer classes, were now less numerous and corresponded with the class gradient observed for other deaths (the great majority). Thus, in 1959–63, 49 of 85 separate causes of death for men, and 54 of 87 for women, were found for which both Classes IV and V had higher SMRs than Class I and II. For only four of the causes as applying to each sex was the opposite found (Black Report, 1980, p. 70). In 1970–72 the comparable number of causes in which, again, both Classes IV and V had higher SMRs than I and II rose, in the case of men, to 68 of the 92 listed — 'which represents a proportionate increase compared with 10 years earlier' (Black Report, 1980, p. 70). For only four causes were mortality ratios for I and II higher than for IV and V: accidents to motor vehicle drivers, malignant neoplasm of the skin, malignant neoplasm of the brain and polyarteritis nodosa and allied conditions (OPCS, 1978, Table 4A).

The class gradient can be examined for 1979–83 for a total of 78 causes and groups of causes. They are listed in Table 9.5a for men aged 20–64 in Britain, showing SMRs for the four occupational classes at the extremes of the dispersion. What are the conclusions which may be drawn from these data? Firstly, the class gradient is more securely established for more causes than in previous decades. For the 78 categories in the list there are 65 where there are higher SMRs for both Classes IV and V than for either Class I or Class II. The reverse applies in only one instance (malignant melanoma of the skin). In eight of the remaining twelve instances (including malignant neoplasm of the colon and of the nasal cavity; malignant

133

Table 9.5a: Standardised Mortality Ratios by cause, rich and poor classes: Great Britain (all men)

		I	II	IV	V
All causes		66	76	116	165
I	INFECTIOUS & PARASITIC DISEASES	65	62	117	215
	Respiratory TB inc late effects	32	35	128	279
	Other TB inc late effects	28	41	120	214
II	NEOPLASMS	69	77	117	154
	Malignant neoplasms (MN)	69	77	117	154
	MN of lip, oral cavity & pharynx	61	73	120	204
	MN of digest. organs & peritoneum	80	83	115	141
	MN of oesophagus	80	77	114	151
	MN of stomach	50	67	127	158
	MN of colon	114	99	101	116
	MN of rectum, etc	88	90	112	139
	MN of pancreas	79	90	117	127
	MN of nasal cavity, m. ear, sinus	43	92	89	208
	MN of larynx	39	63	141	210
	MN of trachea, bronchus & lung	43	63	126	178
	M. Melanoma of skin	133	126	89	82
	Other MN of skin	52	76	130	142
	MN of prostate	77	104	97	109
	MN of bladder	80	77	122	134
	MN of brain	119	98	96	119
	MN of lymph & haematopoietic tissue	107	97	104	121
	Hodgkin's disease	91	89	106	132
	Leukaemia	110	90	106	122
	Lymphoid leukaemia	113	87	108	134
	Acute lymphoid leukaemia	137	97	98	91
	Chronic lymphoid leukaemia	98	82	111	162
	Myeloid leukaemia	114	90	108	124
	Acute myeloid leukaemia	118	90	108	108
	Chronic myeloid leukaemia	106	93	108	155
Benign neoplasms		89	78	87	127
III	ENDOCRINE, NUTRITIONAL ETC, DISEASES	72	76	118	156
	Diabetes mellitus	67	76	123	155
IV	DISEASES OF BLOOD	86	79	98	114
	Anaemias	55	61	117	134
V	MENTAL DISORDERS	35	48	97	342
VI	DISEASES OF NERVOUS SYSTEM	69	61	109	185
	Multiple sclerosis	121	69	110	114
VII	DISEASES OF CIRCULATORY SYSTEM	69	80	113	151
	Chronic rheumatic heart disease	66	71	122	154
	Hypertensive disease	56	66	125	190
	Ischaemic heart disease	70	82	112	144
	Acute myocardial infarction	71	83	111	143
	Diseases of pulmonary circulation	70	71	130	171
	Other forms of heart disease	67	75	116	183
	Cerebrovascular disease	62	72	117	179
	Diseases of arteries & arterioles	82	94	102	119
	Phlebitis, venous emb. & thrombosis	51	70	123	191

Table 9.5a: *contd.*

VIII	DISEASES OF RESPIRATORY SYSTEM	36	50	129	210
	Pneumonia	33	50	121	211
	Bronchitis, emphysema & asthma	34	48	133	211
	Asthma	60	80	128	146
	Pneumoconioses, etc	16	18	240	130
IX	DISEASES OF DIGESTIVE SYSTEM	67	79	112	204
	Ulcer of stomach & duodenum	39	55	124	261
	Gastric ulcer	28	55	127	278
	Duodenal ulcer	45	56	120	253
	Hernia of abdominal cavity	74	52	86	211
	Chronic liver disease & cirrhosis	79	103	106	182
X	DISEASES OF GENITOURINARY SYSTEM	43	69	116	185
	Nephritis & nephrosis	45	72	117	180
	Infections of kidney	30	63	104	248
	Hyperplasia of prostate	65	70	138	103
XII	DISEASES OF SKIN	142	88	115	111
XIII	MUSCULOSKELETAL DISEASES	62	75	111	136
	Rheumatoid arthritis, exc. spine	73	59	125	138
XIV	CONGENITAL ANOMALIES	67	70	105	119
XVI	ILL-DEFINED CONDITIONS	48	43	106	276
XVII	EXT. CAUSE INJURY & POISONING	67	70	121	226
	Transport accidents & late effects	67	80	120	177
	Motor vehicle accidents	65	79	118	181
	Other transport accidents	85	95	141	133
	Accidental poisoning & late effect	47	56	11↑	340
	Accidental poisoning by drugs, etc	43	57	105	337
	Other accidental poisoning	52	56	118	344
	Accidental falls & late effects	57	46	137	277
	Suicide & self-inflicted injury	89	80	114	198
	Open verdicts	52	55	127	304

Source: OPCS (1986) 1979–83 Decennial Supplement.

neoplasm of the prostate; malignant neoplasm of the brain and of the lymph and haematopoietic tissues; leukaemia and lymphoid leukaemia; myeloid leukaemia; multiple sclerosis and diseases of the skin), the combined SMR for Classes IV and V is higher than for combined Classes I and II, and in the other four the SMRs are very nearly equal. In some cases the numbers of deaths on which SMRs are based are very small. Thus, six deaths because of disorders of the skin produced an SMR of 142 for Class I. Indeed, large variations in the number of deaths by cause have to be watched in developing any analysis. The seven causes identified as being exceptions to the standard class gradient account for only 2.9 per cent of the deaths classified for these four years.

Table 9.5b: Standardised Mortality Ratios by cause, rich and poor classes: Great Britain (all women)

		I	II	IV	V
All causes		69	78	110	134
I	INFECTIOUS & PARASITIC DISEASES	66	80	111	153
	Respiratory TB inc late effects	67	57	123	179
	Other TB inc late effects	50	87	162	199
II	NEOPLASMS	87	92	107	117
	Malignant neoplasms (MN)	87	92	108	117
	MN of lip, oral cavity & pharynx	47	96	107	156
	MN of digest. organs & peritoneum	87	89	111	114
	MN of oesophagus	61	75	126	146
	MN of stomach	76	79	118	139
	MN of colon	106	99	100	88
	MN of rectum, etc	77	90	118	125
	MN of pancreas	91	87	108	109
	MN of nasal cavity, m. ear, sinus	23	84	80	155
	MN of larynx	34	42	128	225
	MN of trachea, bronchus & lung	48	69	126	149
	M. Melanoma of skin	118	107	88	98
	Other MN of skin	93	68	102	221
	MN of female breast	109	104	99	94
	MN of uterus	38	69	119	171
	MN of cervix uteri	29	60	124	186
	MN of body of uterus	68	101	108	126
	MN of ovary & other uterine adnexa	103	103	104	99
	MN of bladder	60	69	114	118
	MN of brain	123	104	86	93
	MN of lymph & haematopoietic tissue	91	102	107	107
	Hodgkin's disease	88	102	102	155
	Leukaemia	91	106	101	107
	Lymphoid leukaemia	55	111	74	95
	Acute lymphoid leukaemia	51	99	83	130
	Chronic lymphoid leukaemia	68	130	68	54
	Myeloid leukaemia	95	105	103	106
	Acute myeloid leukaemia	106	101	102	111
	Chronic myeloid leukaemia	72	118	102	94
	Benign neoplasms	85	97	96	118
III	ENDOCRINE, NUTRITIONAL ETC, DISEASES	46	54	116	186
	Diabetes mellitus	45	54	119	191
IV	DISEASES OF BLOOD	71	75	102	125
	Anaemias	112	86	92	75
V	MENTAL DISORDERS	50	57	83	144
VI	DISEASES OF NERVOUS SYSTEM	76	68	96	99
	Multiple sclerosis	109	80	95	79
VII	DISEASES OF CIRCULATORY SYSTEM	90	63	122	158
	Chronic rheumatic heart disease	63	51	122	185
	Hypertensive disease	32	51	115	185
	Ischaemic heart disease	43	58	124	161
	Acute myocardial infarction	41	58	125	159
	Diseases of pulmonary circulation	67	59	111	158

Table 9.5b: *contd.*

	Other forms of heart disease	55	65	112	148
	Cerebrovascular disease	59	71	122	148
	Diseases of arteries & arterioles	49	81	120	145
	Phlebitis, venous emb. & thrombosis	58	62	112	137
VIII	DISEASES OF RESPIRATORY SYSTEM	37	53	115	160
	Pneumonia	39	51	107	138
	Bronchitis, emphysema & asthma	34	55	122	170
	Asthma	43	78	114	128
	Pneumoconioses, etc	136	46	52	130
IX	DISEASES OF DIGESTIVE SYSTEM	58	74	96	148
	Ulcer of stomach & duodenum	41	48	109	205
	Gastric ulcer	48	40	108	209
	Duodenal ulcer	35	51	107	205
	Hernia of abdominal cavity	79	71	113	215
	Chronic liver disease & cirrhosis	60	92	85	109
X	DISEASES OF GENITOURINARY SYSTEM	39	57	116	187
	Nephritis & nephrosis	56	62	111	204
	Infections of kidney	7	43	113	188
XI	COMPLICATIONS OF PREGNANCY, ETC	87	84	136	148
XII	DISEASES OF SKIN	39	53	111	164
XIII	MUSCULOSKELETAL DISEASES	80	73	104	92
	Rheumatoid arthritis, exc. spine	96	59	122	83
XIV	CONGENITAL ANOMALIES	77	53	86	96
XVI	ILL-DEFINED CONDITIONS	73	63	74	126
XVII	EXT. CAUSE INJURY & POISONING	65	79	93	121
	Transport accidents & late effects	84	95	98	109
	Motor vehicle accidents	83	94	97	112
	Other transport accidents	100	131	119	25
	Accidental poisoning & late effect	59	73	103	145
	Accidental poisoning by drugs, etc	54	72	111	139
	Other accidental poisoning	74	78	83	149
	Accidental falls & late effects	47	63	101	111
	Suicide & self-inflicted injury	78	83	83	95
	Open verdicts	44	69	100	156

Source: OPCS (1986) 1979–83 Decennial Supplement.

For women (Table 9.5b) 82 causes or combined causes of death are listed. In 62 of these the SMR is higher for both Classes IV and V than for either Class I or Class II. The reverse applies in four instances (malignant neoplasm of the breast and of the brain, malignant melanoma of the skin and acute lymphoid leukaemia). In a further six instances the SMRs of Classes IV and V, when combined, are higher than of combined Classes I and II. In the remaining ten instances there is no marked gradient either way.

Secondly, the class gradient is much steeper for some diseases than for others. Examples are malignant neoplasm of the larynx and of the trachea, bronchus and lung, respiratory diseases, ischaemic heart disease, cerebrovascular disease and motor vehicle accidents. The causes of death with a shallow class gradient include malignant neoplasm of the colon and of lymph and haematopoietic tissue, leukaemia, diseases of the blood, diseases of the arteries and congenital anomalies. Systematic comparison of such cases should allow causal factors to be identified more exactly.

Thirdly, explanations of the phenomenon plainly have to be rooted in wide ranging and not only specific causes. To concentrate on particular causes of death, without noting their proportionate importance or drawing clues from factors which are implicated in a wide number of causes, may be to overlook major scientific possibilities of prevention as well as cure. In the current discussion, smoking is frequently invoked to illustrate differences in health between classes, with the implication that behaviour patterns under an individual's own control produce these social differences in mortality. Smoking is of course important in causing or precipitating a variety of illnesses, including heart diseases and respiratory diseases, as well as lung cancer, but its place in a total picture of population health, and how it needs to be understood, deserves sophisticated analysis. Thus, for instance, even with malignant neoplasm of the trachea, bronchus and lung (lung cancer), which is linked more strongly with smoking than any other cause, considerable care is needed in interpreting the evidence. Firstly, and to place lung cancer in the context of all deaths, it is worth noting that between 1979 and 1983 it accounted for 11 per cent of all male deaths and well under 5 per cent of all female deaths. Secondly, without underestimating the primary importance of smoking, we should not ignore other contributory factors, which include work conditions, dampness and warmth of housing, the kind of home heating realistically available, air pollution, and facilities and income for exercise. Thirdly, it is not sufficient to lay the blame for smoking at the door of the individual alone. Institutional encouragements and discouragements (including the roles respectively of commercial advertising and education at school) also play a part in the complex aetiology of this disease.

In a paper coinciding with the publication of the most recent decennial supplement, Marmot and McDowall (1986, pp. 274–6) combined all manual and non-manual occupations to overcome the difficulties of mis-classification listed in the OPCS report. They standardised SMRs for 1970–2 to the 1979–83 data. They analysed data for cancer of the trachea, bronchus and lung, coronary heart disease, cerebrovascular disease and all causes of death combined. 'Despite the general fall in mortality the relative disadvantage of manual compared with non-manual classes has increased for each of these 4 cause groups' (ibid., p. 274). In the case of lung cancer they found that for men, mortality had declined more rapidly among non-manual than manual classes. Women's mortality had declined among non-manual but increased among manual classes. The 'social-gradient has widened'. In their view a wider range of causal factors needed to be considered, including unemployment, a widening gap in income between classes and 'environmental/occupational exposures', in addition to differentials in certain aspects of life-style, like diet, alcohol consumption and smoking.

9.1 THE PRESENTATION OF THE EVIDENCE

The national evidence of a high correlation between premature mortality and social or occupational class in the 1980s is therefore very strong. It seems, however, to be treated equivocally in the OPCS report, for reasons which begin with the meanings attributed to 'social class' and the use of the concept latterly by the Registrar General and his staff.

Historically social class has been shown to be a powerful source for the scientific explanation of variations in ill-health and especially mortality. In 1842 William Farr constructed the first English Life Table (Registrar General, 1842) and later a 'Healthy District Life Table' based on 63 districts recording the lowest death rates, which represented a striking contrast with the table for the country as a whole (Farr, 1860). This provided a standard by which 'the loss of life under other circumstances may be measured'. Subsequently, life tables were prepared by statisticians for the rich and prosperous, and differences in expectation of life between the rich and the masses, especially in infancy, came to be measured. In 1887 the Assistant Registrar General addressed the Royal Statistical Society and appealed for the construction urgently of 'the rates of mortality prevailing in the different strata of society' (Humphreys, 1887). He pointed out that the Registrar General of Ireland had already analysed 1881 Census returns for Dublin in terms of four social classes. In 1911 Stevenson responded to scientific and public requests and ranked the population of England and Wales into five social classes (though three groups — namely, miners, textile workers and agricultural workers — were considered to be important enough to pick out separately). From that time onwards successive Registrars General refined and extended the practice, especially in the decennial supplements on occupational mortality. There was never any question but that social class was generally accepted as a phenomenon causally related to measures of ill-health. The classification of occupations was recognised to be important to the understanding of society and social behaviour, and has been regularly updated.

This is not to deny the misgivings sometimes expressed about the relatively crude procedures which were adopted to categorise the population by class. As the Black Research Working Group pointed out, the use of occupation happened to be a convenient means of constructing a classification but left other features of social class unexplored (Black Report, 1980, p. 14). In addition to occupation, a variety of factors may be said to play a part in determining class: income, wealth, type of tenure of housing, education, social origins, family and local connections and style of consumption. These are inter-related with class position or status but none of them can be treated as a sufficient indicator of that position or status. Populations are not found to divide uniformly into different and distinct ranks when graded by income, wealth, housing and access to education, even when there is a high degree of correspondence between positions in the different ranks. Between different periods of a society's history, or between different societies, the number of classes, and the ease with which boundaries may be identified, may change; but that does not contradict the existence of a class structure, any more than the existence of different military structures contradicts the existence of a well-defined military hierarchy of officers and other ranks. To follow the Black Report, 'social classes may be said to be segments of the population sharing broadly similar types and levels of resources, with broadly similar styles of living and some shared perception of their collective condition' (ibid., p. 13).

Occupation has proved to be a remarkably accurate indicator of class in recent British history, at least for the great majority of the population. Thus, it designates not just *type* of work, but likely working conditions (indoors or outdoors, and exposure to dust, noise, dangerous machines, etc.), and likely access to certain facilities or amenities of work as well as fringe benefits. It also provides an approximate guide to likely level of income, because earnings have always accounted for the great bulk of the disposable incomes of families (although, with the development of social security and a retired as well as student class, exceptions and qualifications have grown in importance). As an indicator, however, it seems to be less powerful in the 1980s than it has been in the past. Thus, sociologists have pointed out the difficulties of determining class from the 'general standing' of different occupations, especially during a period when pay and conditions may be varying more widely within as well as between occupations. In addition, more women are in work than in the past and the occupation of male wage-earners is less indicative of the whole family's or household's class (and resources) than once it was. The Black Research Working Group discussed the issue and made a number of positive recommendations which had the effect of maintaining the importance of ranking the population by social class but sought a more effective development of individual 'occupational' class (using objective criteria) and of family class (using information about the occupations of adults in the family and their social class origins) (ibid., pp. 12–20).

The scientific argument has been distorted in the latest decennial supplement (OPCS, 1986). Objections are expressed to the concept of social class by the Registrar General and his colleagues without any attempt to confront or to explore in detail the scientific evidence of a profound correlation between class and mortality for the 1979–83 data as much as the data in all previous decades. The authors of the OPCS report say that

understanding of the causal factors of many diseases has increased to the point where differences in mortality by broad social groups is of limited relevance. This is reflected in the greater emphasis on occupational rather than class mortality differentials in the present study (ibid., p. 17).

Non-scientific examples or references are given to justify the epithet of 'limited relevance'. Moreover, if the difference in mortality between the *combined* occupations falling into different classes is becoming more marked, then this would suggest that factors *common* to different occupations (Low or high pay? Risk of unemployment? Access to property and fringe benefits? Differential changes in working conditions and amenities?) are becoming *more* rather than less important, and factors unique to single occupations of subordinate, or at least lesser, importance.

The authors' second objection to the use of the concept is that

141

'interesting' mortality gradients 'are now seen not to apply to women (when classified to a social class on the basis of their own occupation)' (ibid.). It is certainly the case that when married women are classified by husbands' occupations there is a more consistent gradient of SMRs than when classified by their own occupations. It may be that this is due partly to the variation by class in the number of such women holding part-time employment, or in the number who have been in such occupations for long durations. Again, if incomes, housing and environment are substantially implicated in the higher mortality of poorer classes, then it would not be surprising if male occupations (of longer duration as well as higher earnings than of employed married women) are more representative indicators of the overall class of families than female occupations. The evidence, however does not support the authors' belief that mortality gradients do not apply to women. Some of this is displayed in the text of the OPCS report. Inequalities in mortality (as measured by SMRs) between Classes I and II, on the one hand, and IV and V, on the other, are pronounced in the case of single women and (if the tiny number of deaths in Class I is ignored) all women in the longitudinal study as measured by their own occupations (OPCS, 1986, p. 26). The same is true for single women in all age-groups (ibid., microfiche Table GD19).

The third objection to the concept given by the Registrar General and his colleagues is very unclear. They say that 'the major use of social class in the present study is to try and separate way of life from occupational influences on mortality' (ibid., p. 17). They therefore greatly restrict the interpretation of the concept, and, having so restricted it, they continue, 'however, it cannot be expected that social class, determined in this way from occupation, could account for more than a small part of the influence of way of life on mortality' (ibid., p. 17). The terms are neither precisely defined nor illustrated from the data. Social class is not conceived in a form generally understood in the social sciences. The image in the authors' minds seems to include occupational factors which are restricted to the kind and nature of the work rather than the incomes, the material conditions made possible by those incomes, and the modes of behaviour developed as a consequence over successive lifetimes.

Reservations are also expressed in the report about the 'serious bias' in the calculation of SMRs for social classes (ibid., pp. 17 and 44). However, these are found to apply principally to a category of labourers and unskilled workers not elsewhere classified in social

Class V. The whole of Class V represents only 6 per cent of the male population. No effort appears to have been made to correct for the identified bias and therefore to reproduce all the most important tables in the main printed report. Nor does there seem to have been much disposition to consider how far such reservations apply as much or almost as much to the previous decennial exercises as to the present one without detracting more than marginally from their useful results. As expressed in an editorial in the *Lancet*, there are grounds for the Registrar General's concern about the problems of classification

> but his conclusion that it makes the social class data 'useless' is quite unreasonable. It is vitiated by his chief medical statistician's approval of the concurrent publication of a very useful analysis of time-trends in mortality differentials between grouped aggregates of social classes. If he approves this publication . . . [i.e. Marmot and McDowall, 1986] he should have included at least some presentation of this highly important material within the Decennial Supplement itself (*Lancet* editorial, 1986, p. 611).

In view of the reservations about groups within the smaller Class V, it is therefore regrettable that advantage was not taken in the OPCS report on occupational mortality of presentations combining Classes IV and V, making up about one quarter of the population, and comparing them with Classes I and II (like those, for example, in the Black Report, 1980, and Adelstein and Fox, 1978).

The unwillingness to present data for several decades is also regrettable in view of the admission that the effects of re-classifying occupations on comparisons between the mortality data for 1979–83 and those for 1970–2 'are generally small' (OPCS, 1986, p. 45). There is a further technical point, which illustrates the negative attitude in the report towards social inequality. If the *technical* difficulties of operationalising class so that trends in unequal mortality can be traced are substantial, why was an alternative not developed — for example, using deciles or quintiles? It would have been inexpensive to reconstruct the statistic accordingly and, indeed, to reconstruct the data for previous decades so that trends in mortality could be discerned more clearly and established beyond doubt.

It is difficult not to interpret the Decennial Supplement of July 1986 as an equivocal document, pouring cold water on analyses of social class in the printed commentary in Part I and yet allowing the results of those analyses to be found (with great difficulty and only by having to transpose some data) within the large number of 22,000 tables on microfiche in Part II. The total cost of the 1986 Report is £55.20, which restricts it to the hardiest specialists. Moreover, the means of extracting useful data depends not just on having access to a microfiche display unit but one with a printer as well. ''The virtual absence of any text tables shows a regrettable insensitivity to the needs and interest of that much larger number of readers who do not work in departments of statistics'' (*Lancet* editorial, 1986, p. 611).

The equivocation about social class is nicely symbolised on p. 43 (OPCS, 1986). A table of estimates of ·social class SMRs is published prominently but a note to the table states that 'these data are subject to serious bias and do not represent usable estimates of mortality by social class'. If they were unusable why print them? Perhaps because, deep down, the Registrar General's staff know they are a vital part of the analysis. The categorisation is admittedly crude but provides approximate representation of the structural inequalities which exist in society.

Many specialists will be examining the OPCS data in greater detail. Occupational status as a surrogate for social class has been convenient for administrators and social scientists alike. Now that many women have been employed for long periods of married life, and have themselves contributed to family incomes, and now that more people have the chance of inheriting wealth, especially a house, male occupational status is no longer as powerful a guide to the family's economic position or living standards as it once was. Means have therefore to be found (as the Black Research Working Group argued) to augment occupational status as a basis of identifying social class, perhaps by using objective supporting measures of income or perhaps by combining men's and women's occupations in some form of weighted 'family' class. However, the authors of the latest Decennial Supplement on occupational mortality should reflect that social class is not disappearing or becoming impossible to measure; it merely needs to be measured, even roughly, by alternative or additional means from those traditionally adopted.

This discussion carries a further implication. The social distribution of income and wealth in Britain has become more polarised in the 1980s (indicated by statistical data on earnings, taxation, household incomes, and employment published by different Government departments). The growth of unemployment, together with the relative increase in prematurely retired people, disabled people and one-parent families, and the decline in low-wage levels, has

144

contributed to the growth in numbers of people experiencing hardship. Current statistical studies of inequality in health by area and by class reflect some of the outcomes of that development. Much more work needs to be done on the relationship between the level of life-time resources (both income and wealth) and ill-health, mortality and development. There are relatively few studies. A Canadian study in the Hamilton region, using sophisticated techniques, found that median family income explained nearly half the mortality variation among the census tracts of the study area (Liaw, Hayes and McAuley, 1986). In Britain the work of Wilkinson (1986a, b, see also Carr-Hill, 1985) require replication and expansion elsewhere.

9.2 THE NORTH IN RELATION TO NATIONAL TRENDS

This chapter has presented the recent official evidence about inequalities in mortality, and has gone on to discuss how far that evidence deserves to be accepted publicly as a basis for action. We have concluded that with certain reservations the evidence is emphatic. In the words of a *Lancet* editorial 'Social class inequalities for men, and probably also women, have widened since the 1950s, both relatively and absolutely; and they are now probably greater than at the start of the century' (*Lancet* editorial, 1986, p. 611).

How do inequalities in mortality in the Northern Region compare with those for Britain, or England and Wales, as a whole? Table 9.6 shows that mortality is higher in all classes among both sexes in the

Table 9.6: Mortality of men and women by occupational class, Britain and the Northern Region (SMRs, 1979–80, 82–3)

Occupational Class	Men aged 20–64			Women aged 20–59		
	Britain	Northern Region		Britain	Northern Region	
			as % of UK			as % of UK
I	66	72	109	69	65	94
II	76	83	109	78	83	106
III$_N$	94	106	113	87	92	106
III$_M$	106	115	108	100	103	103
IV	116	138	119	110	129	117
V	165	186	113	134	155	116

Note: Single women classified on own but married women on husband's occupation.
Source: OPCS, 1986, Tables GD38 and GD41.

Table 9.7: Numbers of observed and expected deaths by occupational class, Northern Region, 1979–80, 1982–3

Occupational Class	Men aged 20–64			Women aged 20–59		
	Observed	Expected	'Excess'	Observed	Expected	'Excess'
I	530	733	− 203	161	249	− 88
II	2886	3487	− 601	1097	1318	− 221
III$_N$	1900	1789	111	756	823	− 67
III$_M$	8411	7326	1085	2408	2332	76
IV	5360	3891	1469	1650	1284	366
V	3186	1714	1472	726	469	257

Source: OPCS, 1986, Tables GD38 and GD41.

Table 9.8: Mortality of men and women in different regions of Britain, 1979–80, 1982–3

Region	Direct age-standardised death rate (per 1000)		
	Men 20–64	Single women 20–59	Married women 20–59
Central Clydeside	7.86	1.78	3.23
Strathclyde	7.14	1.66	3.06
North	6.43	1.56	2.50
North West	6.37	1.69	2.52
Remainder of Scotland	6.13	1.47	2.58
Wales	5.86	1.43	2.34
Yorks and Humberside	5.83	1.48	2.32
West Midlands	5.72	1.54	2.26
East Midlands	5.28	1.40	2.14
South East	4.88	1.29	1.97
South West	4.82	1.32	1.93
East Anglia	4.37	1.14	1.79
Scotland	6.92	1.62	2.89
England and Wales	5.43	1.41	2.17
Britain	5.57	1.43	2.23

Source: OPCS, 1986, Tables GD19, GD23 and GD27.

North, with the exception of women in Class I. The table also shows that inequality tends to be greater among both sexes. Standardised mortality is about 17 per cent higher in Classes IV and V in the North than elsewhere in Britain. Table 9.7 turns the Northern rates into estimates of excess deaths. It can be seen that for the four years over the period 1979–83 during which deaths were analysed, there were approximately 4,000 more deaths among male manual workers aged 20–64 and 700 among female manual workers aged 20–59 than

Table 9.9: Mortality of men aged 20–64 and married women aged 20–59, direct age standardised mean annual death rates (per 1,000 population), 1979–80, 1982–3

Social Class	Britain		Northern Region	
	Per 1000	Numbers of deaths	Per 1000	Numbers of deaths
MEN				
I	3.75	(10,808)	4.02	(530)
II	4.25	(56,535)	4.64	(2886)
III$_N$	5.29	(33,370)	5.97	(1900)
III$_M$	5.97	(116,218)	6.44	(8411)
IV	6.51	(69,415)	7.70	(5360)
V	9.44	(36,574)	10.55	(3186)
Armed forces	9.60	(1902)	10.67	(54)
Unoccupied	8.06	(10526)	6.93	(581)
MARRIED WOMEN				
I	1.45	(3532)	1.30	(161)
II	1.81	(17518)	1.98	(1097)
III$_N$	2.04	(8420)	2.16	(756)
III$_M$	2.29	(32,609)	2.36	(2408)
IV	3.04	(17,958)	3.67	(1650)
V	3.99	(7194)	4.50	(726)
Armed forces	1.12	(526)	1.49	(10)
Unoccupied	0.90	(2319)	0.91	(1577)

Note: Married women classified on husband's occupation. Note that the number of deaths given for married women in the Northern Region in fact covers deaths of all women.
Source: OPCS, 1986, Tables GD19 and GD27.

would have been the case if national death rates had applied to these classes. Correspondingly there were some 700 fewer male and 400 fewer female deaths among non-manual workers.

Table 9.8 brings out the North's relative position among regions in Britain. The Northern Region has the third worst male and fourth or fifth worst female death rate. What effect that has on death rates is shown in Table 9.9. Like Table 9.7, this shows the unfavourable experience of all classes, with the exception of women in Class I. Inequalities in health are much sharper in some regions of Britain than in others. When the two most and least prosperous classes are grouped and compared, the North stands out as the region with the widest difference, as Table 9.10 indicates, and this applies to both women and men. This difference deserves to attract considerable scientific and policy interest.

Table 9.10: SMRs for all causes, 1979–80, 1982–3 by region (men aged 20–64 and women aged 20–59)

Standard region county	Men			Women		
	I & II	IV & V	IV & V as % of I & II	I & II	IV & V	IV & V as % of I & II
North	81	152	188	80	136	170
Wales	79	144	182	79	125	158
Scotland	87	157	180	91	141	155
North-West	83	146	176	86	135	157
Yorkshire & Humberside	79	134	170	78	120	154
West Midlands	75	127	169	77	113	147
South-East	67	112	167	71	100	141
East Midlands	74	122	165	73	110	151
South-West	69	108	156	70	96	137
East Anglia	65	93	143	69	81	117
Great Britain	74	129	174	76	116	153

Note: SMR for all men, and for all women, in Great Britain in 1979–80, 1982–3 is 100. Regions ranked by SMR for Classes IV and V combined as a proportion of SMR for Classes I and II combined. Women classified on own or husband's occupation.
Source: OPCS, 1986, Microfiche Tables GD38 and GD41.

Table 9.11: Trends in male mortality in the North, 1970–2 to 1979–80 and 1982–3 (men aged 25–64: all causes)

SMRs for Class I and II combined and Classes IV and V combined

Years	I and II	IV and V	IV and V as a percentage of I and II
1970–2	98	156	159
1979–83	81	153	189

Notes: SMR for all men in Britain in 1979–83 is 100. The 1970–2 figures were standardised with the 1979–83 rates.
  The boundaries of the Northern Region were redrawn in 1974. The Region 'lost' a population of 275,000 to North Yorkshire, and 'gained' a population of 110,000 from Lancashire and the West Riding of Yorkshire which is now in Cumbria.
Sources: OPCS, 1986 (and unpublished tables provided by OPCS); and OPCS, 1978.

Finally, Table 9.11 pulls together the heart of this analysis and illustrates the reasons for present concern. The standardised mortality of the poorest quarter of the population of the North has declined only marginally in the last decade but that of the most prosperous quarter has substantially declined. As a consequence the 'divide' in terms of health has become much greater in what is a very short span of time.

9.3 CONCLUSION

The latest evidence published by the Registrar General confirms widening inequality in the death rates of different social or, more exactly, occupational classes. That inequality has grown sharply both in Britain generally and especially in the Northern Region in the last ten years. It applies both to men and women and is revealed emphatically when the two most prosperous classes are combined and are compared with the two poorest classes. These two each comprise one-quarter of the total population. Wider inequality also applies to more causes of death. For men a 'class gradient' exists for 65 of 78, and for women 62 of 82, categories of death by cause. The reverse applies in only one and four cases respectively. This evidence is not highlighted in the Registrar General's 1986 published report on occupational mortality — although it can be derived from the microfiche tables published with that report, and *is* picked out in major respects in a paper published independently by the retiring principal author of that report. These points are discussed above.

Why does the Registrar General appear to be equivocal about stating the evidence and drawing the implications of that evidence? We have reviewed the technical reasons given by the Registrar General and his colleagues for doubting analysis by occupational or social class. While agreeing that there are distinct problems, they are little different in principle from those arising in previous decades, and can be largely overcome in constructing generalisations about trends. The majority of social scientists appear to agree with this view.

A more worrying reason for failing to highlight the evidence appears to be the disbelief of some influential people in the existence or severity of inequality, and their distrust of the concept of 'social class' not because of any reasoned doubts about its empirical or scientific basis but because of its presumed role in challenging political orthodoxies. We would wish to reaffirm its value as a necessary scientific concept. Occupational or social class is a structural reality throughout the world and has to be used as one of the principal scientific categories explaining social behaviour. It

149

should not be necessary to re-assert such a principle in the late 1980s, but the pedantic objections to the concept of class are being used to divert attention from important developments in the health of the population.

10

Conclusions

This book aims to contribute to the scientific understanding and explanation of inequalities in health in Britain, partly by reviewing recent national evidence about mortality but mainly by examining detailed statistical evidence for small areas covering a major region of the country. For the populations of 678 wards throughout the Northern Region of England the book explores the meaning and practicable measures of 'material deprivation' and 'poor health' and demonstrates a consistent and very strong association between the two.

The publication of the Black Report in 1980 provided emphatic confirmation that the years since the establishment of the National Health Service had not seen a decline in social inequalities in health in Britain. Indeed, it produced evidence of widening inequalities and not just vivid statistical illustrations of big differences in health experience. Perhaps partly fuelled by the Government's dismissive response to that report, and faced with the implications for health posed by the deepest economic recession since the 1930s, public and scientific interest in health inequalities has continued to grow during the 1980s. The swelling number of papers on the problems of resource allocation for health care and area studies of health are just two relevant examples. The present study epitomises this recent development, and provides, perhaps for the first time, an analysis of the health of small areas across an entire region of the country.

The Northern Region is not a microcosm or reflection of the country as a whole, either in health or social and economic terms: rather, it is one of its most deprived constituent parts. The areas of highest mortality and morbidity in Britain are overwhelmingly to be found in the North and North-West, in Scotland and in Wales; they are almost entirely absent from southern England, except for one or two areas of inner London. These are also areas where the recession and its human dimension of unemployment and reduced living standards have been felt most severely. An analysis of inequality in health in the North is, therefore, biased towards the worse end of the health spectrum in Britain, as we showed in the early part of this book.

10.1 AIMS AND CONCEPTS

The study has had two principal aims: firstly, to find ways of depicting the severity and distribution of both poor health and material deprivation — particularly across hundreds of areas within a single region; and secondly, to help to account for the unequal distribution of health by studying its association with material deprivation in particular but also with occupational class.

The first step has been to clarify the key concepts and to select practicable measures for study and analysis. Poor health must be understood as more than a risk of premature death and as more than the prevalence of clinically ascertainable disease. However, in dealing with other features of poor health, it has to be admitted that there is a lack of practicable measures of reduced vitality or activity, discomfort or pain, debility or low morale among the population — to give different examples. At this stage of the analysis of health, it nonetheless seems important to symbolise the principle that scientists must deal with more than mortality experience, even when they include mortality as a necessary datum. Three measures were chosen in this report as examples of this broader approach to the meaning of poor health, namely:

(1) *Mortality*. SMRs for persons (i.e. both sexes together) aged under 65 years, based on deaths over a three-year period, 1981–3.
(2) *Disablement*. The proportion of all residents in private households aged 16 and over who classed themselves as permanently sick or disabled at the 1981 Census.
(3) *Delayed Development*. The proportion of live births below 2,800 gm, based on births over three years, 1982–4.

These three measures have been described separately and in combination, in the form of an 'Overall Health Index'. Analysis of poor health has focused both on the separate and the combined measures.

A coherent conceptualisation of deprivation is equally important.

Material deprivation needs to be separated in principle from social deprivation and then represented, so far as possible, by a sufficient 'spread' of sub-elements or measures which do not simply reproduce or overlap each other and hence misrepresent the reality being measured. A distinction must also be drawn in favour of direct experience of deprivation and not just membership of a sub-group or minority at risk of that deprivation. The incompatibility, duplication and poor coverage of indicators appears to be a problem with much of the scientific study of deprivation at the present time. In this research the following variables were each drawn from the 1981 Census. As discussed in the text, each was independently validated in regression analyses, and in combination provided a much more powerful explanatory variable than any separate component.

(1) *Unemployment*. The percentage of economically active residents aged 16–59/64 who were unemployed.
(2) *Non-ownership of a car*. The percentage of private households not possessing a car.
(3) *Non-ownership of a home*. The percentage of private households renting rather than owning or buying a home.
(4) *Overcrowding*. The percentage of private households containing more than one person per room.

The four separate measures of deprivation were combined to form an 'Overall Deprivation Index'.

10.2 FINDINGS

What were our principal findings? Firstly, the differences in health between local populations are very wide and perhaps more consistently wide than presumed in recent scientific discussion. Different examples can be given. According to the chosen indicators the ward with the poorest overall health was Wheatley Hill in Easington. With a population of 3754 the ward had 52 deaths of persons under 65 and 23 low-weight births in three recent years, and there were 145 people reported as permanently sick or disabled in 1981. At the other extreme, with a roughly comparable population of 4,014, the ward of Hutton in Langbaurgh had 11 deaths and 9 low-weight births and there were only 18 reported as permanently sick or disabled in 1981. Standardised Mortality Ratios (SMRs) and rates worked out on the appropriate population basis are shown for all 678 wards in Appendix 6. The ward with poorest health (Wheatley Hill) had three times as many people unemployed, more than ten times as many households without a car, more than fifteen times as many overcrowded households and twelve times as many households not owning their homes as in the ward of comparable size with best health, namely Hutton.

Although there are pockets of ill-health to be found in every district in the North, there are certain major concentrations of poor health to compare with more dispersed areas of good health. Thus, for example, very high rates of premature mortality were found across a large number of adjoining wards on the south side of the Tees in Middlesbrough and Langbaurgh and in a smaller area straddling the Tyne in Newcastle and Gateshead. The severity of poor health in Easington and Hartlepool is also particularly striking: no less than six of Easington's wards feature among the 25 wards out of the total of 678 with the worst overall health in the Region. Another method of demonstrating inequalities is to compare wards divided into ten or five bands or groups on different criteria. When all 678 wards were divided into ten groups ranked according to SMRs, the 10 per cent with worst mortality had an SMR of 165, compared with an SMR of 58 for the 10 per cent with the lightest mortality (Table 6.5). The ratio between the two is 2.8:1.

The wards were also divided into five groups according to their overall health. The fifth (136 wards) with poorest health had an SMR for persons aged 0–64 of 143 compared with 80 for the fifth with best health. There were 18 per cent of low-weight births in the worst fifth, compared with 10 per cent in the best fifth, and nearly three times as many residents aged 16 and over who were permanently sick and disabled in that fifth of wards with worst overall health. Moreover, through all five ranked bands of wards there was a clear step-wise gradient. This was also true for the available indicators of deprivation.

One graphic illustration of inequalities in health is provided by the two groups of 136 wards each at the top and bottom of the ranking by overall health. In the group of 136 wards with the best health (with a population of 376,000) the SMR is 80, the proportion of people permanently sick is 1.3 per cent and the proportion of low-weight births is only 10.1 per cent. On this basis we can then calculate the 'excess' mortality and morbidity in the 20 per cent of wards with worst health. If the low rates of ill-health had been experienced by the population of 788,000 who live in the 136 wards with the poorest health, then there would have been 1,356 fewer deaths of people under 65 each year; there would have been 13,823 fewer people permanently sick or disabled; and there would have been 890 fewer low-weight live births each year. Such statements can be used to formulate and clarify national and regional health objectives. They can be converted into definitions of attainable objectives in the development of future national health policies.

The second principal finding was that across the spectrum of wards in the Region, variations in health tended to correspond closely with variations in material deprivation or affluence. In other words, whilst the contrast between the extremes of the regional distribution of health and deprivation illustrates most dramatically the argument that a strong association exists between the two, even in the middle ranges of the regional distribution it is apparent that slight variations in social and economic well-being have parallels in slight variations in health. The association between poor health and material deprivation is statistically highly significant, with a correlation of 82 per cent between the Overall Health Index and the Overall Deprivation Index, and is relatively consistent. The different measures of health are also highly inter-correlated (though the measures of mortality and permanent sickness more so than of either of these two when matched with low birthweight). The different measures of deprivation are also highly inter-correlated, and that association is explored in various stages of the analysis above.

One part of the analysis centres on the concept of class, as made operational in the Registrar General's occupational classification (see Chapter 7). Having presented evidence for occupational class gradients in mortality and low birthweight in wards at either end of the health spectrum, an attempt is made to explain how actual patterns of mortality differ from those which might be predicted on the basis of the occupational class composition of the populations of local areas, and how much of the high mortality in the two predominantly urban counties of the Region may be explicable solely in terms of the class structure of those areas.

In practice it was unfortunately impossible to standardise for age and class simultaneously; nevertheless, the indications are that in areas of high mortality a large number, but by no means all, of the additional or 'excess' deaths may be attributed to the occupational class structure. There are also significant variations between one area and another. Most of Sunderland's raised mortality would seem explicable in terms of occupational class composition. In contrast, North Tyneside's high mortality is only to a small degree explained by occupational class composition alone.

These examples help to show that occupational class alone does

155

not uniformly reflect the distribution of mortality: either there are factors independent of occupational class which contribute in substantial measure to any further explanation of excess deaths; or occupational class includes systematic variations in the experience of material deprivation which need to be revealed if a further large number of the observed excess deaths are to be explained. Another way of expressing this point is that occupational class is an imperfect representation of social class. If that is true then a substantial number of individuals will have been in effect misallocated to the wrong 'social' class. This leads to a second stage of our further analysis, in which the deprivation variables are reintroduced into the discussion, and are examined to discover how much of the variation in health they severally and in combination 'explain'.

What were already strong associations between individual measures of poor health and deprivation were found to become stronger when they were replaced by the combined measures — that is, the Overall Health and Overall Deprivation Indices. The strongest of the associations obtained was that between permanent sickness or disability and material deprivation. As is inevitable among a large number of local populations, there were interesting paradoxes. Areas with similar levels of severe deprivation sometimes differed significantly in health. Middlesbrough and Sunderland provide the most clearcut illustration of this, both districts containing large numbers of extremely deprived wards: but whilst in Middlesbrough these highly deprived wards for the most part experience ill-health which places them amongst the very worst in the region, in Sunderland the most deprived wards consistently experienced significantly less bad — though certainly by no means good — health. Regression analysis has been used to assess how much of the variation in health in certain groups of wards can be explained in statistical terms.

All four of the components of the Overall Deprivation Index make a significant contribution to explaining the variation in overall health. However, when individual counties are compared, different patterns emerge. The forms of deprivation with greatest explanatory value, and the extent to which they can explain the variance in health, are by no means identical in the five counties and the patterns are discussed in some detail in the text. Among the four deprivation indicators, only car ownership, the one which seems best to reflect relative material affluence, stands out in the regression equations for all five counties.

In each county the four deprivation indicators explain more of the variation in health than any of the indicators based on occupational class. Perhaps that is because they are closer to reflecting material economic standing in the community. Even when occupational class is incorporated into an extended set of deprivation measures, any improvement in accounting for variations in health is at best marginal. In other words, the explanatory power of the four deprivation variables is shown to be considerable — thereby justifying their initial choice.

In a final analysis, concentrating on mortality in Cleveland and Tyne and Wear, the regression technique is used to show how far actual mortality differs from that predicted on the basis of the experience of deprivation in each area. Mortality was higher in South Tees and especially central Tyneside than knowledge of the deprivation experienced in these areas would seem to imply. In contrast, mortality was relatively lower in North and West Sunderland.

Pollution has not figured in our operational measures of material deprivation. This problem needs to be remedied in future research, and depends upon producing measures which can be applied to small areas. It seems likely that the particular industrial configuration of the Teesside basin, and of factors operating in areas along the Tyne, and associated consequences of long-term exposure to various forms of environmental pollution, may be an important additional influence contributing to the high mortality in these areas. Given the limited sources of data available, the possibility can be no more than raised. We hope it will be followed up rigorously.

At the end of July 1986, the long-heralded OPCS report on occupational mortality was published. That report is equivocal about the value of analyses by social class but incorporates (especially in microfiche available with the 'Commentary' in Part I) mortality data which demonstrate both the relatively worse mortality of the Northern Region and the widening national health gap between sections of the population ranked high and low on the social scale. In a special analysis of the microfiche tables issued with the OPCS report in July 1985, we compared trends in rates of mortality for occupational Classes I and II (now 27 per cent of the population) with those for Classes IV and V (now 29 per cent of the population). The change since the late 1940s is unmistakeable. Relative to the poorer classes the mortality rates of the richer classes have substantially diminished since 1949. For men and women aged 25–34, the rates of Classes I and II in the early 1980s were less than half what they were in 1949–53. Rates of Classes IV and V have also

157

diminished at the younger adult ages, but not as quickly. In middle age, however, there is now a striking difference. In 1979–83 the male mortality rate in England and Wales for those aged 45–54 in Classes IV and V was only 7 per cent lower, and for those aged 55–64 only 3 per cent lower than in 1949–53, whereas the rates in the richest classes had diminished by 37 per cent and 33 per cent respectively. The trends among women were similar, though the differences were a little less sharp.

At the beginning of Chapter 2 we referred to the work in the 1930s by M'Gonigle and Kirby (1936). This documented the social inequalities in health existing within Stockton-on-Tees and within Newcastle upon Tyne. Such inequalities persist today — between North and South, between the professional and managerial classes and the semi-skilled and unskilled classes, and between wards within each of the towns and cities in the North. This last point needs emphasising: the differences in levels of deprivation or privilege between wards in each town and city in the North are generally mirrored by differences in the health of their populations. Fifty years after M'Gonigle and Kirby were writing, the situation they described still exists.

In September 1984 the British Government joined all other European member countries in endorsing a World Health Organization Regional Office for Europe strategy. The primary aim was a reduction in inequalities in health by 25 per cent by the year 2000. The present study has documented just how great are the present inequalities in health within one severely deprived region of Britain.

Notes

1. In a recent study of relative prosperity in British local labour market areas, four of the six least prosperous areas were in the Northern Region (Champion and Green, 1985).
2. This is the case on both the Department of Environment's 'Basic' or 'Economic' Z-scores.
3. The wards making up these clusters are as follows:

(a) *South Tees Area*: Victoria, Ayresome, St Hilda's, Gresham, Southfield, North Ormesby, Grove Hill, Berwick Hills, Park End, Pallister, Thorntree, South Bank, Church Lane, Grangetown, Coatham;
(b) *Central Tyne Area*: West City, Moorside, Bensham, Bede, Deckham, Felling;
(c) *North Tyne Area*: Scotswood, Benwell, Elswick, Moorside, West City, Sandyford, Byker, Monkchester, Walker, Walkergate, Wallsend, Howdon, Riverside;
(d) *Easington and East Durham Area*: Sherburn, Shadforth, Cassop cum Quarrington, Coxhoe, Fishburn, Old Trimdon, New Trimdon, Deaf Hill, Thornley, Wheatley Hill, Wingate, Hutton Henry, Shotton, Passfield, Howletch, Dene House, Acre Rigg, Eden Hill, Horden South, Horden North, Easington Village, Easington Colliery;
(e) *Whitehaven and Cleator Moor Area*: Sandwith, Mirehouse West, Mirehouse East, Hensingham, Cleator Moor North, Cleator Moor South, Frizington.

4. Blue Hall estate is the focus of a recent study of health and deprivation in two neighbouring but contrasting areas of Stockton (Marsh and Channing, 1986).
5. Exact comparisons between Cleveland and Tyne and Wear local unemployment rates since the 1981 Census are not possible because different population bases are used in the two counties. Cleveland figures are from Cleveland County Planning Department.
6. The wards making up this cluster in Sunderland are: Castletown, Town End Farm, Southwick, Colliery, South Hylton, Grindon and Thorney Close.

Glossary

Black Report: The Report of the Government Working Group on Inequalities in Health, known as the Black Report because its Chairman was Sir Douglas Black, formerly Chief Scientist at the Department of Health and President of the Royal College of Physicians. The other members of the Group were Professor J.N. Morris, Dr Cyril Smith and Professor Peter Townsend.

Morbidity: Illness

OPCS: Office of Population Censuses and Surveys. The arm of the Government Statistical Service which is in charge of the national Census and many other recurrent and occasional surveys and collections of statistics.

Registrar General: The head of the OPCS. The current Registrar General is Mrs G.T. Banks.

Registrar General's Decennial Supplements: The OPCS publishes mortality and morbidity data annually. Every ten years it supplements these annual publications with extra information from the ten-year Census and publishes two Decennial Supplements, one on occupational mortality and the other on area mortality.

Registrar General's Social Classes: A system of classifying individuals (and their dependants) on the basis of their present occupation (or previous one, in the case of unemployed people). There are five social Classes (I–V), Class III being further split into IIIM (manual) and IIIN (non-manual). The Registrar General's social class classification was introduced in 1911 to help analyse variations in demographic statistics in general, and infant mortality statistics in particular.

SMR: Standardised Mortality Ratio. SMRs are calculated to enable mortality comparisons between different areas to be made after taking account of their different age/sex population structures — that is, one area can be compared with another after holding age and sex constant. Standardisation is usually to the mortality experience of England and Wales as a whole, and an area whose mortality is no worse or better than that of England and Wales would have an SMR of 100. Thus, the Northern Region with an SMR of 112 in 1985 experiences worse mortality than England and Wales even allowing for its different population structure. An SMR may cover deaths at all ages or just those in a certain age range, for example ages 0–64. SMRs may sometimes be produced after standardising for an area's occupational class structure in addition to its age/sex structure.

Appendices

1. DATA SOURCES, DEFINITIONS OF THE VARIABLES AND HANDLING THE DATA

A. Data sources

This study has been made possible by the recent availability of three sets of data: the 1981 Census Small Area Statistics, postcoded death registration records, and postcoded birth registration records. All of these data are provided by the Office of Population Censuses and Surveys. The ward is the smallest viable area (in England and Wales) for analysis using Census data and postcoded data, and the accuracy of assignments of births and deaths to a ward depends on the correctness of the postcode which has been given at the time of registration, and on the quality of the OPCS Postcode Directory which has been used to assign postcodes to wards. OPCS estimate that births and deaths are assigned to wards with about 95% accuracy. Variables have been produced for each of the Region's 678 wards as constituted on 1 January 1984. One hundred and ninety-eight of these wards have been created following boundary changes since the 1981 Census; for these wards the original Census data was re-assembled.

B. Definitions of the variables

(i) *The health variables*

The three health variables which are combined to form the Overall Health Index are:

  (a) *Permanent sickness*: the percentage of all residents aged 16 and over in private households who classified themselves as permanently sick or disabled at the 1981 Census;

  (b) *Premature mortality*: the standardised mortality ratio for deaths between 0 and 64 years inclusive, produced by relating a ward's mortality experience in 1981–3 inclusive of its population at the 1981 Census, and standardising to

163

the experience of England and Wales over the same period;

(c) *Low birthweight*: the percentage of live births under 2,800 gm during 1982–4 inclusive. (This period, rather than 1981–3, was chosen because only since 1982 has the recording of birthweight been virtually 100 per cent.)

(ii) *The deprivation variables*

The four main deprivation variables, which are the components of the Overall Deprivation Index, and the additional socio-economic variables have all been produced from the 1981 Census Small Area Statistics.

C. Handling the data

To cater for the presence in some wards of institutions such as mental hospitals, the deprivation variables have been calculated so as to refer only to people resident in private households. By excluding from the analysis 1,666 deaths of people aged 0–74 who died in an institution after a stay of six months or more, or in one which was considered to be their home, we have made the SMRs refer as far as possible only to people resident in their own home. The analysis is based on registrations in 1981–3 of 58,059 deaths of people aged 0–74.

2. THE CREATION OF SUMMARY VARIABLES:
THE Z-SCORE TECHNIQUE

The well-established Z-score technique has been used to produce the
two summary variables, the Overall Health Index and the Overall
Deprivation Index. Two of the deprivation variables — those
relating to unemployment and overcrowding — were firstly
transformed using the log transformation $y = \ln(x + 1)$ to produce
more Normal distributions.

For each variable the mean and standard deviation are:

Variable	Mean		Standard Deviation	
HEALTH				
Permanent sickness	2.33		1.01	
Low birthweight	13.95		4.10	
Persons 0–64 SMR	109.27		31.01	
DEPRIVATION				
Unemployment	11.72	(2.42)	6.56	(0.51)
Lacking Car	42.01		17.58	
Not Owner Occupied	50.10		22.77	
Overcrowding	3.31	(1.36)	2.01	(0.45)

(Figures in brackets are values of the transformed variables)

3. ESTIMATING THE NUMBER OF DEATHS DUE TO AN AREA'S OCCUPATIONAL CLASS STRUCTURE

The number of deaths expected in an area's male population aged 15–64, on the basis of its occupational class structure, has been calculated by applying England and Wales's mean annual crude death rates for each occupational class to those men economically active. For those men who are not economically active we have assumed an occupational class distribution the same as that for the economically active men in the same area.

The most recent published data on death by occupational class for men in England and Wales related to deaths of men aged 20–64 in 1979–80 (Source: OPCS, Titchfield, May 1985). To produce similar rates for the male population aged 15–64, these rates were scaled down to reflect the fact that the crude death rate of men aged 15–64 is less than that for men aged 20–64. Thus, the rates used in the analysis were

Occupational Class	Mean Annual Crude Death Rate for Men 15–64, 1979–80
I	0.00293
II	0.00387
IIIN	0.00484
IIIM	0.00507
IV	0.00695
V	0.00969

We would place caveats on the results of this part of our analysis for the following reasons:

(1) It was not possible to take account of different age distributions in the different classes, because the necessary data are not available;

(2) Occupational class death rates for the economically inactive were not available and we have had to assume that this group is subject to the same mortality as the economically active. In practice the result of this may be to underestimate the mortality of the economically inactive since this group will contain many who are permanently sick and therefore subject to greater mortality rates.

4. URBAN AREAS: DEFINITION

Urban areas containing populations over 20,000 people are defined as follows:

(a) *Tyne and Wear*: Entire county

(b) *Cleveland*: Hartlepool
Teesside — consisting of
    Billingham
    Eston and South Bank
    Middlesbrough
    Redcar
    Stockton
    Thornaby

(c) *Cumbria*: Carlisle
Barrow and Isle of Walney
Kendal
Whitehaven
Workington

(d) *Durham*: Durham
Bishop Auckland
Chester-le-Street
Consett
Darlington
Newton Aycliffe
Peterlee
Seaham
Stanley and Annfield Plain

(e) *Northumberland*: Ashington
Blyth
Cramlington

Source: OPCS, 1984

5. ADDITIONAL TABLES AND FIGURES

Figure A5.1: Unemployment. Proportion of each district's population living in wards ranked among the best and worst fifth in the Northern Region

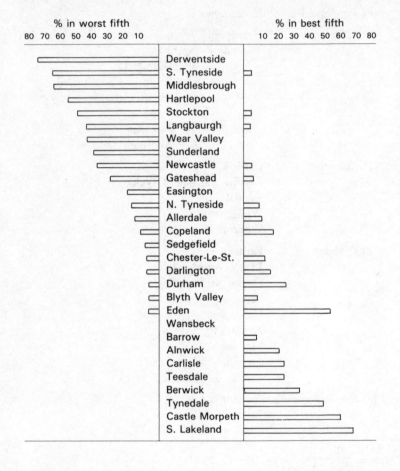

Note: Districts are ranked on the basis of the proportion of population in the worst fifth of wards.

Figure A5.2: Car ownership. Proportion of each district's population living in wards ranked among the best and worst fifth in the Northern Region

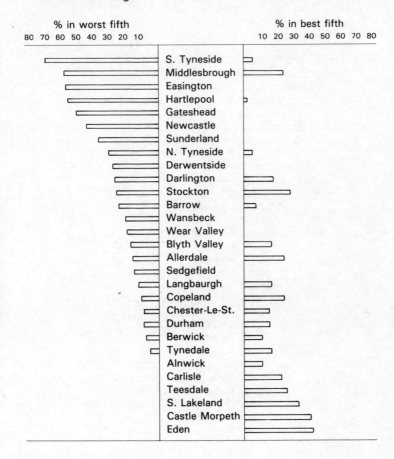

Note: Districts are ranked on the basis of the proportion of population in the worst fifth of wards.

Figure A5.3: Overcrowding. Proportion of each district's population living in wards ranked among the best and worst fifth in the Northern Region

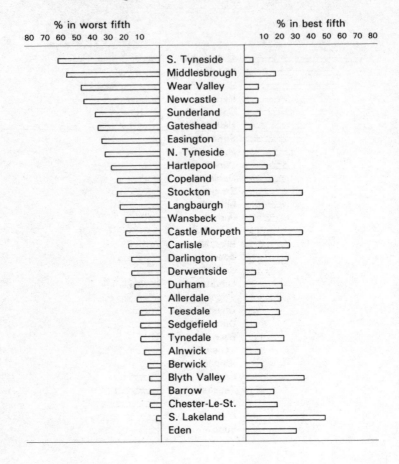

Note: Districts are ranked on the basis of the proportion of population in the worst fifth of wards.

Figure A5.4: Home ownership. Proportion of each district's population living in wards ranked among the best and worst fifth in the Northern Region

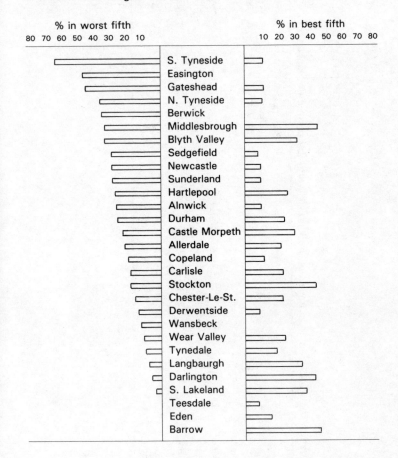

Note: Districts are ranked on the basis of the proportion of population in the worst fifth of wards.

Table A5.1: Health and deprivation for ward groupings based on ranking of wards by permanent sickness

	Worst health decile (68 wards)	Best health decile (68 wards)	Ratio Worst/Best
Residents 16 + permanently sick (%)	4.2	0.9	4.7
Persons 0–64 SMR (actual number of deaths)	138.8 (4382)	86.8 (1184)	1.6
Live births under 2,800 gm (%)	16.6	11.6	1.4
Unemployed persons 16–59/64 (%)	20.4	5.5	3.7
Households not owner-occupied (%)	77.7	22.8	3.4
Households with no car (%)	65.4	20.2	3.2
Households with more persons than rooms (%)	5.7	1.3	4.4

Table A5.2: Health and deprivation for ward groupings based on ranking of wards by low birthweight

	Worst health decile (68 wards)	Best health decile (68 wards)	Ratio Worst/Best
Live births under 2,800 gm (%)	20.7	7.2	2.9
Residents 16+ permanently sick (%)	3.3	1.7	1.9
Persons 0–64 SMR	134.9 (3166)	91.0 (1196)	1.5
Live births under 2,500 gm (%)	9.3	3.4	2.7
Infant mortality (deaths under one year per 1000 live births)	13.3	8.3	1.6
Unemployed persons 16–59/64 (%)	18.0	7.8	2.3
Households not owner-occupied (%)	66.0	31.8	2.1
Households with no car (%)	59.4	29.6	2.0
Households with more persons than rooms (%)	5.7	1.8	3.2

Table A5.3: Health and deprivation for ward groupings based on ranking of wards by persons 0–64 SMR

	Worst health quintile (136 wards)	Next quintile (136 wards)	Middle quintile (134 wards)	Next quintile (136 wards)	Best health quintile (136 wards)
Persons 0–64 SMR (actual deaths)	150.4 (8520)	123.4 (7093)	109.3 (6337)	94.0 (4250)	70.9 (1942)
Live births under 2,800 gm (%)	16.7	15.2	14.2	13.5	12.4
Residents 16+ permanently sick (%)	3.3	2.9	2.4	2.0	1.7
Infant mortality rate	12.4	11.0	8.7	9.4	9.3
Male 0–14 SMR (actual number of deaths)	135.7 (337)	101.1 (231)	76.6 (181)	77.2 (142)	81.0 (97)
Female 0–14 SMR (actual number of deaths)	125.9 (227)	116.5 (192)	93.1 (160)	79.1 (107)	71.9 (60)
Male 15–44 SMR (actual number of deaths)	131.8 (654)	106.7 (527)	97.5 (506)	87.5 (361)	80.1 (202)
Female 15–44 SMR (actual number of deaths)	134.4 (359)	105.1 (291)	96.3 (285)	79.6 (191)	72.2 (106)
Male 45–64 SMR (actual number of deaths)	153.1 (4357)	127.5 (3671)	114.5 (3245)	95.9 (2124)	65.9 (889)
Female 45–64 SMR (actual number of deaths)	156.9 (2586)	127.6 (2181)	113.6 (1960)	99.4 (1325)	74.0 (588)
Male 65–74 SMR (actual number of deaths)	128.7 (4498)	118.6 (4479)	110.7 (4125)	105.7 (3113)	92.7 (1681)
Female 65–74 SMR (actual number of deaths)	126.7 (3028)	114.9 (2952)	108.5 (2775)	104.0 (2079)	97.7 (1187)
Unemployed persons 16–59/64 (%)	19.7	15.1	12.0	9.7	7.7
Households not owner-occupied (%)	68.9	58.6	51.0	39.3	34.9
Households with no car (%)	62.4	53.5	46.5	37.9	29.5
Households with more persons than rooms (%)	5.7	4.2	3.2	2.5	2.0

Note: Actual number of deaths in parentheses.

Table A5.4: Selected avoidable deaths[a]. SMRs for deaths between 0–64 years for ward groupings based on ranking of wards by persons 0–64 SMR for all causes (numbers of deaths in parentheses)

Cause and sex (ICD 9th Revision Codes)		Worst mortality quintile (136 wards)		Best mortality quintile (136 wards)		Ratio Worst/Best
Malignant neoplasm of cervix uteri (180)	F	182	(81)	65	(15)	2.8
Chronic rheumatic heart disease (393–398)	M	188	(29)	67	(5)	2.8
	F	230	(61)	69	(9)	3.3
Hypertensive disease (401–405)	M	107	(29)	53	(7)	2.0
	F	150	(21)	88	(6)	1.7
Cerebrovascular disease (430–438)	M	164	(299)	66	(58)	2.5
	F	163	(243)	56	(41)	2.9
Pneumonia and bronchitis (480–486, 490)	M	179	(162)	55	(24)	3.3
	F	147	(93)	36	(11)	4.1
Asthma (493)	M	151	(26)	60	(5)	2.5
	F	169	(30)	125	(11)	1.4
All avoidable deaths[b]	M	160	(592)	62	(112)	2.6
	F	167	(572)	61	(103)	2.7

Notes: a. These categories were selected because in the Region as a whole there were more than 50 deaths per year from each disease.
b. for the full list of avoidable deaths see the footnote to Table 6.6.

Table A5.5: Avoidable deaths in Tyne and Wear and Cleveland: SMRs for the worst quarter of wards in each district for deaths between 0–64 years, 1981–3 inclusive

District	SMR (number of deaths in parentheses)	
Hartlepool	202	(52)
Stockton	198	(81)
Middlesbrough	195	(69)
Gateshead	173	(82)
Langbaurgh	172	(47)
Sunderland	167	(112)
South Tyneside	147	(67)
Newcastle upon Tyne	150	(83)
North Tyneside	121	(67)

Note: The full list of avoidable deaths, with ICD 9th Revision Codes, is Tuberculosis (010–018, 137), Malignant neoplasm of cervix uteri (180), Hodgkin's disease (201), Chronic rheumatic heart disease (393–398), Hypertensive disease (401–405), Cerebrovascular disease (430–438), Appendicitis (540–543), Cholelithiasis and Cholecystitis (574–575.1), Pneumonia and bronchitis (480–486, 490), Asthma (493), Acute respiratory disease (460–466, 470–474), Abdominal hernia (550–553), Bacterial infections (004, 037, 320–322, 382–384, 390–392, 680–686, 711, 730), Maternal deaths, (630–678), Deficiency anaemias (280–281).

Table A5.6: Relationships within the two sets of variables: Spearman rank correlation coefficients (678 wards)

(a) HEALTH

		1	2	3
Persons 0–64 SMR	1	1.00		
% residents 16+ permanently sick	2	0.53	1.00	
% live births under 2,800 gm	3	0.37	0.40	1.00

(b) DEPRIVATION

		1	2	3	4
% unemployed 16–59/64	1	1.00			
% households overcrowded	2	0.74	1.0		
% households with no car	3	0.83	0.74	1.00	
% households not owner-occupier	4	0.52	0.65	0.63	1.00

Note: All of the above correlation coefficients are highly statistically significant of a strong association.

Table A5.7: The relationship between Overall Health and the deprivation and class indicators in each Northern Region county: Spearman rank correlation coefficients

Deprivation and Class indicators	Overall Health Index					
	Tyne & Wear (113 wards)	Cleveland (98 wards)	Cumbria (171 wards)	Durham (177 wards)	Northumberland (119 wards)	Region (678 wards)
% unemployed	0.80	0.89	0.70	0.64	0.61	0.78
% households with more persons than rooms	0.79	0.83	0.57	0.61	0.44	0.70
% households with no car	0.85	0.89	0.61	0.72	0.71	0.80
% households not owner-occupied	0.80	0.76	0.40	0.60	0.39	0.57
% households with single parent family	0.74	0.83	0.49	0.53	0.50	0.65
% unemployed 16–24	0.76	0.86	0.59	0.59	0.59	0.72
% 17 year-olds not in full-time education	0.78	0.81	0.55	0.61	0.48	0.65
% households with head in Class IV or V	0.86	0.81	0.50	0.59	0.29	0.60
% households with head in Class IIIM, IV or V	0.77	0.81	0.59	0.68	0.60	0.73
Overall Deprivation Index	0.88	0.88	0.71	0.76	0.67	0.82

Note: All of the above correlation coefficients are highly statistically significant of a strong association.

Table A5.8: Regressions of Overall Health Index on deprivation and class indicators for each Northern Region county: proportion of variance in overall health explained by each regression

County	Combination of some or all of the seven deprivation and other socio-economic indicators and the manual Class variable chosen by stepwise regression		Combination of some or all of the seven deprivation and other socio-economic indicators and the Class IV and V variable chosen by stepwise regression	
Region	% households with no car % unemployed 16–24 % 17 year-olds not in full-time education % households overcrowded	66%	% households with no car % unemployed 16–24 % 17 year-olds not in full-time education % households overcrowded	66%
Tyne & Wear	% households with no car % households overcrowded % households not owner-occupied	78%	% households headed by person in Class IV or V % households with no car % households with single parent family	80%
Cleveland	% unemployed 16–59/64 % households with no car	81%	% unemployed 16–59/64 % households with no car	81%
Cumbria	% unemployed 16–59/64 % 17 year-olds not in full-time education % households with no car	51%	% unemployed 16–59/64 % 17 year-olds not in full-time education % households with no car	51%
Durham	% households with no car % 17 year-olds not in full-time education % unemployed 16–24 % households not owner-occupied	61%	% households with no car % 17 year-olds not in full-time education % unemployed 16–24 % households not owner-occupied	61%
Northumberland	% households with no car % unemployed 16–24	53%	% households with no car % unemployed 16–24	53%

Note: The seven deprivation and other socio-economic indicators are % unemployed 16–59/64, % households with no car, % households with more persons than rooms, % households not owner-occupied, % households with single parent family, % 17 year-olds not in full-time education, and % unemployed 16–24.

6. RANKING OF THE 678 WARDS ON THE OVERALL HEALTH INDEX: 1 = WORST HEALTH, 678 = BEST HEALTH

Ward	Local authority	Persons 0-64 SMR	No. of deaths	% Perm. sick	No. Perm. sick	% Low wt. births	No. Low wt. births	Depri-vation rank	Unem-ployed %	House-holds with no car %	House-holds over-crowded %	House-holds owner occpd %	Class IV & V house-holds %
1 Wheatley Hill	Easington	159	52	4.9	145	24.0	23	124	15.3	61.1	3.8	74.7	33.3
2 West City	Newcastle Upon Tyne	191	136	5.1	369	18.6	91	3	29.8	84.3	7.9	97.1	49.5
3 Henknowle	Wear Valley	189	37	4.6	85	20.7	12	146	16.5	58.3	3.4	70.1	26.0
4 Bede	Gateshead	197	147	4.4	314	19.9	87	25	22.7	77.2	6.6	84.6	41.2
5 Woodhouse Close	Wear Valley	167	81	5.4	227	19.8	49	13	23.5	67.0	10.9	86.7	46.0
6 New Brancepeth	Durham	154	18	4.6	51	24.5	12	55	19.0	62.4	7.6	71.8	38.5
7 Portrack & Tilery	Stockon-on-Tees	200	100	5.3	256	15.3	45	48	29.1	70.6	3.9	75.8	41.6
8 Willington East	Wear Valley	127	42	5.1	150	23.7	28	141	16.9	57.7	3.9	67.6	35.4
9 Deneside	Easington	139	59	5.4	204	20.2	35	28	18.5	79.0	5.3	96.7	45.3
10 Shotton	Easington	141	52	7.0	235	13.4	18	87	17.1	63.3	4.8	74.6	42.7
11 St. Hilda's	Middlesbrough	180	57	4.4	128	18.4	46	10	32.9	78.2	9.4	66.8	47.4
12 South Bank	Langbaurgh	193	88	3.6	156	19.3	102	21	34.1	69.1	10.5	59.6	44.3
13 Sandwich	Copeland	211	53	3.6	86	16.8	27	40	18.5	67.9	7.1	79.7	62.9
14 Owton	Hartlepool	182	91	4.1	189	18.3	62	4	29.7	73.2	8.4	95.2	46.9
15 Eden Hill	Easington	169	74	4.7	214	17.7	68	26	22.4	62.9	8.7	90.5	44.8
16 Hartlepool	Hartlepool	179	82	3.4	155	21.4	63	57	28.8	71.4	5.5	55.0	41.7
17 Plawsworth	Chester-le-Street	179	19	3.0	31	23.0	14	127	18.2	49.1	5.5	65.9	32.4
18 Wingate	Easington	169	54	4.4	135	18.3	24	209	12.9	53.0	3.5	66.3	29.3
19 Old Trimdon	Sedgefield	141	41	4.6	119	20.7	25	106	13.2	57.6	4.6	87.0	39.5
20 Craghead	Derwentside	81	21	5.8	144	22.7	25	66	25.9	63.3	5.3	67.5	34.7
21 Howdon	North Tyneside	148	146	4.2	332	20.1	75	43	18.4	71.6	5.2	87.5	37.5
22 Berwick Hills	Middlesbrough	146	90	4.8	206	17.5	32	38	26.1	67.4	5.4	78.4	47.8
23 Horden North	Easington	166	75	4.0	166	18.1	34	214	10.3	61.3	3.6	59.4	32.1
24 Scotswood	Newcastle upon Tyne	160	127	3.8	298	19.6	134	12	26.5	73.7	12.3	68.2	38.8
25 Church Lane	Langbaurgh	170	58	3.4	111	19.6	48	6	28.4	68.2	8.9	91.7	40.5
26 Kendal Highgate	South Lakeland	163	22	2.7	40	23.2	16	177	57.5	57.5	4.4	75.6	22.0

No.	Teams	District												
27	Teams	Gateshead	136	120	4.3	337	20.2	70	30	20.8	73.8	6.9	82.6	43.7
28	Blue Hall	Stockton-on-Tees	150	77	3.1	162	23.1	90	108	23.9	57.9	5.9	50.1	25.0
29	Startforth with Boldron	Teesdale	148	9	1.8	11	28.6	8	650	5.0	23.1	0.3	30.6	30.0
30	Neville	Sedgefield	147	46	3.6	94	21.2	17	263	10.9	44.4	3.2	68.2	25.0
31	South Moor	Derwentside	115	42	4.3	145	22.6	35	149	24.2	58.4	5.7	31.1	38.9
32	Grangetown	Langbaurgh	194	68	3.2	106	16.5	47	14	32.6	69.0	8.6	80.8	54.6
33	Deerness	Durham	130	39	4.3	120	20.3	30	182	16.3	54.1	4.1	57.4	32.5
34	Felling	Gateshead	151	115	3.3	249	21.1	94	7	22.1	72.3	10.8	88.0	37.1
35	Salterbeck	Allerdale	147	46	3.0	80	22.9	32	34	20.1	62.1	6.5	95.3	55.7
36	Tower	Berwick-upon-Tweed	192	38	1.9	37	21.3	23	193	14.2	48.8	3.8	69.6	26.7
37	Southfield	Middlesbrough	167	59	2.9	110	20.5	70	44	27.0	73.4	9.6	38.2	42.6
38	Tow Law	Wear Valley	140	27	3.8	65	20.3	16	152	20.2	53.8	5.2	47.7	38.0
39	Riverside	North Tyneside	159	119	2.9	206	21.2	115	19	25.6	76.3	6.5	84.6	36.9
40	Thorntree	Middlesbrough	175	137	4.0	292	14.6	77	2	36.7	76.6	8.3	95.9	53.9
41	Pallister	Middlesbrough	164	76	3.4	145	18.4	46	1	30.9	76.1	13.4	92.2	54.2
42	Rossmere	Hartlepool	151	83	3.7	172	18.8	41	70	22.5	61.2	4.9	75.6	41.4
43	Newtown	Stockton-on-Tees	130	68	4.0	193	20.3	70	94	23.9	62.8	5.2	55.1	33.1
44	Catchgate	Derwentside	190	48	4.0	93	12.4	19	116	26.6	55.8	4.2	58.8	18.0
45	Thornley	Easington	127	36	4.1	104	20.2	23	121	14.3	59.0	4.4	76.3	41.3
46	Beckfield	Middlesbrough	136	70	3.0	159	22.8	76	53	25.6	63.2	5.0	77.9	34.4
47	South Stanley	Derwentside	127	55	4.5	175	17.6	39	83	24.8	64.0	4.2	66.9	35.6
48	Moorside	Newcastle upon Tyne	162	94	3.5	205	16.9	51	31	17.8	79.1	5.2	92.5	34.1
49	Brus	Hartlepool	148	89	3.4	164	19.0	35	39	19.9	70.8	4.5	92.5	36.2
50	Stanley Hall	Derwentside	139	47	3.7	123	18.9	31	112	22.6	61.2	2.8	77.6	28.1
51	Horden South	Easington	119	38	4.3	130	19.1	29	181	10.2	60.4	6.6	48.5	38.1
52	Hardwick	Stockton-on-Tees	147	57	3.5	148	18.5	60	11	25.9	69.5	7.8	96.4	41.0
53	Crookhall	Derwentside	184	27	2.5	39	17.6	16	207	29.1	52.4	5.2	16.9	42.5
54	Longbenton	North Tyneside	143	136	3.5	264	18.8	82	69	16.0	68.7	4.9	82.0	31.3
55	Deckham	Gateshead	171	122	3.4	245	15.2	66	41	22.3	68.8	6.7	73.0	35.3
56	Park End	Middlesbrough	156	96	3.3	165	17.3	49	17	29.0	64.6	9.1	84.2	50.4
57	Beechwood	Middlesbrough	122	61	4.2	177	18.1	43	20	27.7	69.4	6.7	88.8	52.0
58	Choppington	Wansbeck	137	33	4.0	87	16.8	21	90	15.7	59.2	4.4	85.6	39.1
59	Cornforth	Sedgefield	125	35	4.3	108	17.0	19	171	15.1	57.8	2.6	77.1	44.3
60	New Trimdon	Sedgefield	161	23	4.4	61	11.8	8	269	12.4	48.1	3.7	57.3	31.6
61	Bede	South Tyneside	131	118	4.4	316	15.5	47	27	25.7	72.2	5.2	94.8	37.0

62	Grove Hill	Middlesbrough	166	63	3.0	119	16.6	36	71	25.6	59.7	6.9	56.9	41.0
63	Monkchester	Newcastle upon Tyne	153	123	3.7	271	15.3	60	9	21.1	78.3	8.9	88.7	42.1
64	Central	Wansbeck	169	56	3.3	101	14.5	27	217	9.6	56.1	4.8	56.8	24.4
65	Ayresome	Middlesbrough	167	89	3.6	189	13.4	55	79	24.6	65.6	5.9	52.7	42.6
66	Passfield	Easington	124	22	2.9	61	22.0	36	101	16.9	49.0	4.3	91.9	19.4
67	Wheatbottm & Helmingtn Rw	Wear Valley	128	37	4.7	121	14.0	13	123	17.3	57.2	4.8	66.9	31.5
68	Elswick	Newcastle upon Tyne	131	85	2.9	214	20.8	104	67	18.9	69.5	6.5	62.5	23.0
69	Broom	Sedgefield	110	51	4.2	178	18.3	40	210	14.1	55.0	2.8	67.8	36.1
70	Mandale	Stockton-on-Tees	136	81	3.3	192	18.5	80	115	21.7	52.7	5.6	59.7	39.4
71	Thorney Close	Sunderland	135	139	4.3	401	14.6	55	18	26.3	52.5	5.7	97.3	39.2
72	Pelaw	Durham	139	29	4.1	89	14.9	22	22	22.6	72.3	7.1	89.4	50.9
73	Bensham	Gateshead	148	104	3.4	242	16.4	85	36	21.7	74.7	6.1	73.7	31.6
74	St. Hilda	Hartlepool	150	82	2.9	152	18.1	56	47	25.4	69.1	4.6	77.1	37.7
75	Victoria	Stockton-on-Tees	151	64	2.8	119	18.2	54	185	20.5	59.1	4.5	35.7	26.2
76	Coundon	Wear Valley	126	50	4.0	155	16.7	40	113	18.4	53.8	6.3	60.9	32.1
77	Roseworth	Stockton-on-Tees	105	60	3.5	168	21.5	62	97	21.9	55.8	4.7	71.1	32.7
78	Castletown	Sunderland	138	134	3.5	286	17.1	74	24	22.8	67.1	7.3	93.2	33.6
79	Holborn Hill	Copeland	121	28	2.2	45	24.3	25	317	10.4	60.8	3.7	51.5	25.8
80	Burnhope	Derwentside	78	8	5.4	53	17.0	8	63	26.9	58.3	4.4	81.7	54.2
81	Park East	Darlington	135	64	3.2	146	18.4	66	120	18.8	61.9	6.1	47.4	30.4
82	Easington Colliery	Easington	142	83	3.9	203	14.5	35	178	8.4	58.3	5.3	69.9	23.2
83	Ewanrigg	Allerdale	152	44	3.1	78	16.3	17	46	24.0	62.9	5.5	80.6	45.9
84	Warden & Newbrough	Tynedale	152	12	2.0	16	20.8	5	335	8.3	33.3	3.6	63.0	14.8
85	Alnwick Clayport	Alnwick	104	18	3.4	57	21.4	22	62	16.2	55.6	8.2	81.1	50.0
86	Lascelles	Darlington	132	38	2.5	73	21.2	34	234	11.7	58.1	3.1	57.4	40.2
87	Walker	Newcastle upon Tyne	129	121	3.7	323	16.8	86	5	23.2	81.6	8.6	93.3	41.4
88	Byker	Newcastle upon Tyne	136	97	3.8	265	15.5	45	42	17.1	81.4	3.6	93.5	37.6
89	Newbiggin East	Wansbeck	123	42	3.3	107	19.1	27	156	12.2	59.4	4.5	67.0	36.6
90	Washington North	Sunderland	136	116	3.7	304	15.8	91	92	19.0	59.6	3.9	81.3	30.3
91	Chester West	Chester-le-Street	138	48	4.2	133	13.4	21	82	16.7	61.6	3.3	96.8	43.2
92	Hirst	Wansbeck	156	54	3.3	116	14.7	38	100	15.9	64.2	5.1	68.7	29.3
93	Mirehouse West	Copeland	169	39	1.9	41	18.6	31	29	17.2	58.8	9.5	99.0	46.9
94	Wallsend	North Tyneside	140	118	3.4	260	16.3	71	78	16.8	69.5	4.9	71.8	32.6
95	High Colliery	Easington	153	27	3.3	49	14.9	11	896	13.0	63.6	3.8	96.2	27.5
96	Westbourne	Middlesbrough	157	51	2.7	108	19.3	81	91	24.3	60.1	9.9	29.8	27.8

No.	Ward	District												
97	Collingwood	North Tyneside	121	125	2.6	232	21.8	50	109	13.4	54.5	6.3	76.0	32.7
98	Leam	Gateshead	126	105	2.8	220	20.2	89	45	18.0	60.6	8.2	78.3	30.9
99	South Hylton	Sunderland	123	110	3.6	314	17.4	84	15	27.2	67.4	8.8	86.8	35.0
100	Fawdon	Newcastle upon Tyne	112	111	3.6	316	18.7	91	88	17.8	63.1	5.1	69.7	27.0
101	Cockerton West	Darlington	134	40	2.8	74	18.7	21	126	14.1	59.7	3.2	85.6	22.9
102	Benwell	Newcastle upon Tyne	125	95	3.2	257	18.3	82	51	19.7	71.2	6.6	67.9	29.4
103	Grange	Stockton-on-Tees	157	61	2.3	91	17.6	39	98	19.1	49.6	6.5	70.7	41.9
104	Parkfield	Stockton-on-Tees	130	59	2.9	144	18.7	71	107	22.6	61.9	6.0	46.9	25.2
105	Lumley	Chester-le-Street	149	52	2.6	88	17.4	32	337	9.6	38.3	3.8	48.2	23.5
106	South Hetton	Easington	128	29	3.9	80	14.8	16	239	9.9	59.8	2.3	71.5	22.4
107	Brandon	Durham	110	53	3.2	158	19.8	53	227	11.5	52.3	2.8	71.7	25.0
108	Cornsay	Derwentside	149	20	3.4	41	13.6	9	175	17.9	50.8	3.1	70.4	33.3
109	Southwick	Sunderland	140	127	3.9	328	12.7	54	16	25.1	69.7	9.6	83.0	37.2
110	Hebburn South	South Tyneside	113	80	3.3	182	18.5	28	77	18.4	59.7	4.8	82.9	22.6
111	Dipton	Derwentside	107	23	3.7	85	17.4	19	183	24.1	51.3	3.3	52.3	36.8
112	Plessey	Blyth Valley	146	52	3.0	97	15.2	15	157	15.5	59.1	2.7	77.2	32.1
113	Lockwood	Langbaurgh	158	44	3.6	95	15.2	13	238	17.8	39.5	6.1	35.1	33.3
114	Coxhoe	Durham	128	50	3.6	132	11.0	23	186	10.4	57.4	3.8	72.9	28.6
115	Chirton	North Tyneside	129	107	2.8	216	18.2	63	75	18.9	70.3	4.6	71.7	41.5
116	All Saints	South Tyneside	147	95	2.7	172	16.1	64	56	20.3	70.8	4.8	77.4	30.2
117	Low Sp'moor & Tudhoe Grnge	Sedgefield	127	55	3.1	137	17.1	36	173	16.8	58.3	2.9	67.1	32.1
118	Jackson	Hartlepool	131	61	2.5	120	19.0	64	216	20.2	61.8	4.4	22.1	32.8
119	Blakelaw	Newcastle upon Tyne	127	119	3.3	299	16.2	81	122	14.0	55.9	5.5	71.8	23.6
120	Eastbourne North	Darlington	119	33	2.6	63	20.1	41	150	16.2	54.5	5.3	56.2	27.7
121	Central	Darlington	142	40	3.0	78	15.4	22	155	16.9	54.5	5.6	43.5	39.6
122	Lamesley	Gateshead	128	105	3.9	271	13.6	41	167	13.2	56.2	3.3	73.2	36.0
123	Dyke House	Hartlepool	140	69	2.8	151	16.4	59	60	24.3	58.7	6.8	59.6	45.8
124	Coatham	Langbaurgh	141	43	2.9	92	15.8	29	256	21.7	65.8	2.7	32.0	26.4
125	Ushaw Moor	Durham	144	46	3.7	121	15.8	26	264	11.3	56.8	4.0	54.5	24.5
126	Dene House	Easington	120	39	3.2	108	17.3	32	190	12.7	48.8	3.4	79.5	26.7
127	Wrekendyke	Gateshead	128	109	3.4	255	15.4	48	84	14.9	56.9	6.4	79.4	27.4
128	Cleadon Park	South Tyneside	128	79	3.2	194	15.7	31	52	19.7	65.5	6.6	75.0	34.1
129	Crook South	Wear Valley	131	45	3.5	121	16.4	22	251	15.2	48.3	3.5	49.1	20.2
130	Hetton	Sunderland	117	122	3.9	374	14.5	65	232	12.0	54.8	3.0	62.8	22.4
131	Dunston	Gateshead	137	115	2.8	227	16.5	35	189	12.8	57.9	4.6	55.3	30.6

No.	Area	District												
132	Escomb	Wear Valley	138	19	3.6	53	13.1	13	329	13.3	33.1	5.7	27.3	14.3
133	Tyne Dock and Simonside	South Tyneside	129	65	2.5	115	18.7	51	59	18.9	69.3	5.2	77.6	40.4
134	Kenton	Newcastle upon Tyne	113	116	3.2	280	18.0	85	117	18.7	55.4	5.8	60.5	22.4
135	Ulverston East	South Lakeland	172	22	1.7	22	16.2	13	223	12.1	47.5	5.4	51.6	23.8
136	Town End Farm	Sunderland	134	109	3.0	265	15.9	115	8	26.7	69.2	8.6	92.7	36.2
137	Prudhoe North	Tynedale	127	28	3.4	63	15.2	12	134	9.0	65.2	3.4	87.5	29.8
138	Isabella	Blyth Valley	129	48	2.0	75	20.5	30	148	12.5	54.7	3.6	83.1	32.7
139	Ferryhill	Sedgefield	122	48	3.3	118	16.2	33	246	14.9	54.8	2.9	50.8	35.2
140	Amble East	Alnwick	136	33	3.1	76	15.2	15	151	14.2	57.0	4.3	66.6	26.3
141	Tudhoe	Sedgefield	108	36	3.5	103	17.1	19	200	14.1	53.1	3.5	66.4	36.4
142	Village	Stockton-on-Tees	146	69	2.4	107	16.7	29	270	16.5	42.0	3.9	44.0	31.3
143	Gresham	Middlesbrough	158	61	2.0	87	16.7	69	154	20.5	63.0	7.2	20.6	32.5
144	Framwellgate Moor	Durham	120	38	3.6	109	15.2	15	236	10.1	46.5	4.5	62.6	32.9
145	Esh	Derwentside	103	36	3.7	121	16.8	28	198	12.6	54.9	4.1	62.7	32.3
146	Willington West	Wear Valley	110	26	4.3	105	13.3	15	132	10.8	52.5	5.0	62.4	24.6
147	Mirehouse East	Copeland	129	33	2.2	45	19.3	17	204	10.8	47.0	2.5	96.4	44.3
148	Colliery	Sunderland	121	104	3.2	261	16.1	66	72	19.5	65.5	6.6	62.4	28.4
149	Edward	Berwick-upon-Tweed	181	27	2.7	38	10.1	7	58	13.6	61.3	6.3	93.6	41.7
150	St. Cuthbert's	Stockton-on-Tees	130	59	3.2	143	14.8	33	296	14.2	49.5	2.7	46.6	33.9
151	Blaydon	Gateshead	127	96	3.2	239	15.2	63	135	15.6	60.8	4.0	67.5	30.1
152	Sacriston	Chester-le-Street	122	45	3.3	126	15.4	30	199	14.5	53.5	3.8	61.5	20.9
153	Cleator Moor South	Copeland	152	42	3.0	75	12.6	18	168	13.2	48.9	6.2	59.7	39.7
154	St Cuthbert Without	Carlisle	105	16	2.8	37	19.6	9	508	7.9	19.0	3.4	33.3	16.7
155	Sandyford	Newcastle upon Tyne	131	105	2.7	212	16.5	51	102	16.7	72.5	3.1	71.3	29.9
156	Lingfield	Darlington	134	46	2.6	82	16.5	22	314	11.5	50.3	3.7	43.0	31.9
157	St. Aidan's	Stockton-on-Tees	121	69	2.9	131	17.1	36	172	17.6	53.0	4.1	62.7	30.9
158	Skinningrove	Langbaurgh	111	17	3.4	47	16.3	14	272	19.7	55.4	2.2	16.5	48.6
159	Grangefield	Stockton-on-Tees	110	47	2.5	104	20.0	40	443	12.0	38.6	2.8	19.9	20.7
160	North Road	Darlington	147	42	2.7	73	14.2	24	284	13.1	64.4	5.6	35.1	33.0
161	Boldon Colliery	South Tyneside	121	82	3.1	193	16.0	47	81	15.3	60.7	3.8	80.7	36.0
162	Charltons	Stockton-on-Tees	110	54	3.1	134	17.5	45	93	24.1	63.9	7.3	66.5	38.3
163	Coundon Grange	Wear Valley	127	24	2.7	48	16.9	15	166	19.7	51.6	3.0	32.3	31.0
164	Mile House	Stockton-on-Tees	95	58	3.7	184	16.9	29	96	21.9	62.1	4.0	81.2	38.0
165	Shadforth	Durham	97	13	3.4	44	17.8	13	202	12.7	48.9	4.0	70.0	30.3
166	Sherburn	Durham	143	39	4.0	102	9.2	9	225	9.0	49.3	3.7	75.4	21.7

167	Sunnydale	Sedgefield	126	35	2.1	57	19.0	19	226	11.5	58.0	5.1	40.8	34.2
168	Stanley	Wear Valley	126	18	3.6	48	13.0	7	213	18.0	50.0	6.5	27.4	21.9
169	Broughton	Allerdale	156	21	2.2	27	14.7	10	356	10.7	35.1	2.3	57.3	19.4
170	College	Wansbeck	103	31	2.8	77	19.3	26	294	8.0	57.8	2.4	65.2	28.4
171	Lynesack	Teesdale	121	16	1.9	22	20.5	9	448	9.7	29.3	2.5	32.9	19.4
172	Grindon	Sunderland	117	124	3.1	286	16.1	87	65	21.5	59.7	5.5	79.0	28.6
173	Leadgate	Derwentside	123	45	3.5	117	13.6	18	118	28.6	56.7	4.2	52.7	30.2
174	Hebburn Quay	South Tyneside	127	78	2.9	179	15.5	89	37	22.7	70.2	6.1	76.1	33.0
175	Cramlington East	Blyth Valley	135	55	2.9	107	14.5	29	153	13.8	54.2	3.5	79.1	34.6
176	Rekendyke	South Tyneside	114	70	3.1	176	16.3	51	33	22.1	76.4	5.4	81.9	36.5
177	St Helen's	Wear Valley	117	28	4.3	95	10.9	17	68	23.0	61.4	6.1	67.3	35.9
178	West	Sedgefield	110	48	2.9	136	17.4	56	138	17.7	45.0	3.7	85.4	40.9
179	Chester South	Chester-le-Street	125	52	3.3	113	13.7	13	408	9.1	43.4	1.3	54.2	16.7
180	Primrose	South Tyneside	141	101	2.6	186	14.3	39	64	18.6	60.7	6.5	77.6	30.0
181	Ebchester and Medomsley	Derwentside	128	52	3.0	111	14.5	24	242	21.3	43.9	3.3	45.6	19.1
182	Consett South	Derwentside	119	48	3.5	121	13.5	23	32	41.3	63.1	5.0	76.0	47.8
183	Overfields	Langbaurgh	140	64	2.6	118	14.3	34	119	20.2	49.6	5.0	69.1	32.2
184	Westfield	Allerdale	128	47	2.7	83	15.3	29	80	19.0	60.4	4.8	78.6	39.6
185	Edmondsley	Chester-le-Street	140	7	3.2	16	11.8	4	137	17.4	53.4	4.2	70.3	33.3
186	Brinkburn	Hartlepool	123	56	2.6	117	16.4	48	208	17.7	61.0	4.0	37.7	24.6
187	Flimby	Allerdale	146	23	2.0	27	15.7	11	283	12.1	47.2	3.5	52.4	37.5
188	Evenwood with Ramshaw	Teesdale	95	19	2.6	48	20.0	19	230	13.0	49.3	5.5	42.4	40.7
189	Acre Rigg	Easington	102	32	3.5	107	15.4	24	165	11.7	48.2	4.1	83.7	28.7
190	Aspatria	Allerdale	135	32	2.3	58	15.9	13	338	10.2	45.1	2.3	55.8	28.8
191	High Fell	Gateshead	121	105	3.9	295	11.2	24	23	17.0	69.7	8.8	94.7	36.2
192	Northumberland	North Tyneside	116	93	2.2	167	18.7	89	254	11.7	58.4	3.0	52.5	22.2
193	Chopwell and Rowlands Gill	Gateshead	118	101	3.6	282	12.7	38	233	15.3	53.8	3.6	46.3	27.9
194	Battle Hill	North Tyneside	115	93	2.4	214	17.9	97	222	11.2	48.3	4.9	58.0	10.0
195	North Ormesby	Middlesbrough	140	62	2.7	120	13.3	54	74	24.3	67.9	8.3	39.1	42.3
196	Witton Gilbert	Durham	123	26	3.0	63	14.3	17	349	9.7	38.6	2.8	51.9	21.2
197	Hutton Henry	Easington	123	17	3.3	49	12.9	11	218	17.4	47.7	3.8	52.1	20.9
198	Belle Vue	Carlisle	115	33	2.8	129	16.0	52	266	13.5	46.1	3.9	48.2	23.6
199	Camperdown	North Tyneside	119	94	2.6	210	16.3	69	160	14.5	54.3	3.2	78.5	24.4
200	Fishburn	Sedgefield	112	21	3.3	58	14.3	8	244	10.6	50.6	3.1	67.9	42.6
201	Barrow Island	Barrow-in-Furness	144	40	1.2	35	18.5	39	140	14.2	67.7	5.3	49.3	34.2

202	Thickley	Sedgefield	119	57	2.4	102	16.9	38	95	13.3	62.5	5.9	74.7	38.2
203	Kitty Brewster	Blyth Valley	141	40	2.7	63	12.7	13	219	12.4	51.4	3.5	64.0	27.4
204	Croft	Blyth Valley	124	30	2.3	59	16.7	33	129	18.0	68.5	3.1	64.0	40.2
205	Eppleton	Sunderland	122	119	3.0	280	14.0	58	380	10.7	51.2	3.2	56.6	21.8
206	Holywell	Blyth Valley	95	26	2.3	66	20.4	23	383	9.1	44.1	1.4	59.7	25.8
207	Easterside	Middlesbrough	120	57	3.2	136	13.4	19	49	24.1	62.4	5.6	79.0	32.8
208	Bardon Mill	Tynedale	94	9	2.1	18	21.3	10	597	6.2	23.8	0.8	36.7	20.0
209	Chilton	Sedgefield	114	55	3.2	150	14.1	37	235	14.7	48.8	3.9	50.0	37.9
210	Hendon	Sunderland	136	105	2.6	206	13.6	66	179	29.6	57.1	5.1	37.8	22.5
211	Annfield Plain	Derwentside	88	29	4.0	122	14.2	17	243	33.2	53.8	2.2	45.8	19.7
212	Woolsington	Newcastle upon Tyne	112	89	2.8	221	15.9	73	73	15.4	57.6	7.1	79.1	31.8
213	Northgate South	Darlington	144	40	1.7	48	16.1	28	333	13.2	57.2	2.9	21.8	32.2
214	Crook North	Wear Valley	89	11	3.1	40	17.6	9	286	14.0	50.4	3.6	40.3	26.5
215	St Chad's	Sunderland	116	122	2.9	266	15.0	63	143	16.6	52.6	4.6	66.6	25.7
216	Warnell	Allerdale	101	13	1.6	20	22.2	14	592	5.0	14.7	2.0	33.3	9.8
217	Pelton Fell	Chester-le-Street	77	18	3.7	79	16.8	18	110	16.2	57.5	4.0	83.2	29.4
218	Netherhall	Allerdale	154	33	2.2	46	12.6	11	381	12.1	45.3	1.7	41.1	25.4
219	Upperby	Carlisle	1,11	59	2.8	136	15.8	29	128	13.8	53.8	4.9	76.2	21.4
220	Morpeth South	Castle Morpeth	105	20	1.5	25	22.0	18	437	7.5	36.5	2.5	38.4	20.4
221	Deaf Hill	Easington	94	10	4.5	43	11.1	5	295	12.4	58.5	1.7	57.2	44.4
222	Ryhope	Sunderland	117	115	3.8	372	11.0	64	130	16.5	50.9	5.3	68.7	23.9
223	Ellenborough	Allerdale	143	40	1.9	55	15.2	35	194	14.8	50.5	4.3	60.4	35.2
224	Thorneholme	Sunderland	131	92	1.8	141	17.2	76	274	15.8	55.8	2.7	41.4	19.9
225	Hindpool	Barrow-in-Furness	127	69	2.6	125	14.4	35	316	12.3	63.2	2.5	31.1	38.1
226	Cassop-cum-Quarrington	Durham	111	47	3.2	126	14.1	26	253	10.0	48.2	3.4	67.4	30.0
227	Harton	South Tyneside	116	94	3.0	186	14.0	22	136	17.4	62.4	2.4	80.2	23.4
228	Grange Villa	Chester-le-Street	108	8	3.5	33	13.0	10	169	18.3	52.9	7.3	33.3	43.3
229	Fenham	Newcastle upon Tyne	116	124	2.8	244	14.8	40	245	11.4	58.0	3.1	55.3	17.0
230	Cowpen	Blyth Valley	115	51	3.3	120	12.8	17	50	16.2	64.4	5.5	93.3	46.9
231	Kirkleatham	Langbaurgh	130	69	2.6	146	13.6	40	241	15.4	48.1	2.7	62.0	28.4
232	Pittington & West	Durham	127	34	3.4	91	10.6	12	191	12.2	46.3	5.5	64.4	35.1
233	Bedlington Central	Wansbeck	116	47	3.0	110	13.7	20	273	10.2	51.3	3.4	56.6	27.1
234	St Michael's	Allerdale	136	48	1.8	62	15.9	35	328	12.8	53.3	2.7	33.0	26.3
235	Cockerton East	Darlington	118	56	2.2	94	16.6	32	292	11.2	50.4	3.7	45.0	25.8
236	Bearpark	Durham	86	13	3.2	49	16.7	13	114	10.8	58.9	5.4	82.8	28.2

237	Silloth	Allerdale	112	25	1.9	41	18.4	14	401	10.7	39.2	1.9	42.7	30.9
238	Seton	Berwick-upon-Tweed	173	24	2.7	36	7.1	4	265	9.7	58.1	2.6	62.0	24.3
239	Northgate North	Darlington	156	44	2.0	58	12.2	24	211	15.8	65.8	4.2	32.9	37.1
240	Central	Sunderland	123	115	3.1	289	12.1	82	76	23.8	73.4	4.8	55.4	31.6
241	Saltwell	Gateshead	113	87	2.4	185	16.1	62	158	14.4	62.9	4.0	59.9	27.3
242	Central	Barrow-in-Furness	125	57	2.2	97	15.4	37	299	15.3	61.9	3.4	17.4	29.9
243	Lynemouth	Castle Morpeth	67	13	3.7	62	16.9	10	144	9.0	51.2	4.9	89.7	23.8
244	Ingleby Barwick	Stockton-on-Tees	136	19	0.7	10	20.0	17	667	7.1	6.3	0.3	14.6	9.8
245	Houghton	Sunderland	122	105	3.0	248	12.4	52	197	12.2	52.2	4.4	64.8	25.8
246	Tarns	Allerdale	122	18	1.8	24	17.3	9	539	6.3	18.6	2.1	37.0	20.0
247	Monkton	South Tyneside	110	76	2.9	183	14.2	43	99	17.2	60.3	5.4	68.2	21.9
248	Cockfield	Teesdale	101	17	2.2	32	18.4	9	320	10.8	43.6	3.8	43.5	39.0
249	Eston	Langbaurgh	134	66	2.3	107	13.5	28	184	18.9	47.7	4.6	53.3	34.0
250	Staindrop	Teesdale	98	12	2.0	23	19.4	7	482	7.0	36.2	0.7	60.0	30.8
251	Belford	Berwick-upon-Tweed	98	9	2.3	20	18.2	6	363	8.5	35.1	2.0	69.1	25.8
252	Delves Lane	Derwentside	143	58	3.2	121	8.6	13	103	28.7	52.2	4.3	64.7	29.8
253	Winlaton	Gateshead	111	83	2.9	198	14.0	32	407	9.1	43.3	1.8	44.6	18.5
254	Eastbourne South	Darlington	117	35	2.2	64	15.9	31	89	16.9	61.1	7.3	58.7	29.2
255	Biddick Hall	South Tyneside	102	78	3.0	182	14.7	44	35	19.0	69.4	5.6	93.3	34.1
256	West Auckland	Wear Valley	118	30	2.6	62	14.1	13	302	11.5	42.1	3.8	48.1	35.4
257	Bothal	Wansbeck	117	47	3.0	103	12.6	13	341	6.8	56.6	1.8	63.1	16.7
258	Langley Moor & Meadowfield	Durham	102	19	2.3	40	17.4	15	421	9.4	41.9	1.9	39.6	21.1
259	Stannington	Castle Morpeth	173	18	1.2	12	12.5	4	502	6.0	22.8	1.1	65.6	24.2
260	Ormsgill	Barrow-in-Furness	114	55	2.4	116	15.4	49	285	11.8	55.9	3.7	39.3	27.7
261	Newcomen	Langbaurgh	123	60	2.9	126	12.1	23	104	19.6	51.9	7.3	58.4	24.6
262	Haydon	Wansbeck	73	18	2.7	66	19.3	17	345	8.3	48.9	2.3	54.5	20.0
263	Newbarns	Barrow-in-Furness	95	50	2.0	89	19.3	26	398	9.3	41.8	1.9	45.8	25.2
264	Whiteleas	South Tyneside	136	104	2.9	192	10.2	25	85	15.9	61.0	5.1	80.5	35.2
265	Alston Moor	Eden	117	18	2.4	36	14.7	10	322	18.0	35.9	2.8	43.3	17.8
266	Havannah	Derwentside	99	44	3.6	155	12.2	24	307	16.3	47.8	2.4	42.7	27.9
267	Horsley Hill	South Tyneside	114	97	2.4	165	15.0	35	215	15.2	52.2	3.3	58.1	19.5
268	Shiney Row	Sunderland	103	94	3.6	315	11.6	52	188	12.6	55.7	4.0	64.6	26.1
269	Cleator Moor North	Copeland	140	47	2.0	67	13.2	26	259	12.4	43.0	5.2	46.9	26.4
270	South Tynedale	Tynedale	107	8	1.1	8	21.2	7	451	6.3	14.5	3.1	59.6	24.0
271	Holystone	North Tyneside	108	91	2.3	185	16.1	57	282	10.8	51.0	2.5	65.0	22.0

272	Castle	Allerdale	130	34	1.5	38	16.5	18	573	8.5	28.2	0.8	26.3	13.5
273	Blackhalls	Easington	86	45	3.0	145	16.2	37	301	9.6	52.6	3.6	44.7	19.1
274	Murton East	Easington	101	53	3.0	148	14.2	36	313	8.0	54.2	3.0	54.0	23.9
275	Middridge	Sedgefield	126	36	2.2	79	14.1	42	308	11.8	35.5	2.5	70.3	25.9
276	Park	Wansbeck	128	43	2.8	74	11.4	13	161	9.7	57.7	4.8	74.2	20.3
277	Botcherby	Carlisle	116	58	2.5	114	14.2	40	61	14.2	53.9	8.5	87.3	45.0
278	Seaton	Hartlepool	118	50	2.2	86	15.1	27	483	11.2	29.4	2.1	19.5	24.8
279	St Aidans	Carlisle	121	48	1.7	74	16.7	47	396	8.7	50.7	2.7	25.3	21.8
280	Ryton	Gateshead	116	82	2.8	190	12.8	30	324	9.8	47.0	3.4	45.3	23.0
281	Ulverston Central	South Lakeland	147	20	1.9	24	12.3	8	518	7.4	41.4	1.3	23.3	17.1
282	Clifton	Allerdale	128	20	2.4	34	12.8	10	163	16.2	43.8	4.3	75.5	27.8
283	Woodham	Sedgefield	118	46	2.3	89	14.6	31	298	11.7	36.4	2.3	76.5	33.1
284	Windermere Town	South Lakeland	165	29	1.2	21	12.8	10	350	10.1	42.3	1.9	59.1	21.4
285	Beacon and Bents	South Tyneside	135	80	2.6	149	11.0	37	125	17.9	63.0	4.9	54.7	27.2
286	Chevington	Castle Morpeth	112	28	2.3	59	15.4	16	111	12.2	54.8	6.0	81.0	27.3
287	Harbour	Copeland	114	31	2.4	63	14.7	17	300	10.5	51.8	2.2	61.3	27.5
288	Silksworth	Sunderland	111	102	3.3	313	11.4	50	224	13.7	50.1	3.3	62.0	22.0
289	Grange	Newcastle upon Tyne	90	88	2.4	220	17.7	47	368	8.3	49.8	1.8	53.6	17.3
290	Kirkby Thore	Eden	134	15	1.9	19	14.0	6	445	5.4	22.7	3.6	52.8	34.4
291	Trinity	Carlisle	117	50	2.4	103	14.2	34	331	10.0	53.7	2.7	42.1	21.0
292	Birtley	Gateshead	115	75	3.2	213	11.1	33	276	10.9	49.0	3.7	53.3	25.7
293	Ullswater	Eden	89	9	1.7	15	20.6	7	554	6.4	19.0	1.4	42.1	16.7
294	Middlestone	Sedgefield	98	42	2.5	97	16.0	29	237	13.0	45.2	4.5	53.8	28.6
295	Walkergate	Newcastle upon Tyne	99	94	3.0	275	13.8	58	196	13.7	58.9	5.0	46.1	19.7
296	Eggleston	Teesdale	45	3	2.0	12	25.0	9	564	5.7	13.4	2.9	26.0	4.5
297	Risedale	Barrow-in-Furness	104	49	2.4	101	15.7	45	220	14.2	58.1	4.1	43.9	27.4
298	Spittal	Berwick-upon-Tweed	110	26	1.5	36	18.5	20	229	9.5	50.1	3.2	76.8	25.0
299	Maswell	Easington	74	11	4.5	61	10.9	7	162	14.4	47.4	4.7	72.1	40.0
300	Preston	Stockton-on-Tees	92	19	1.7	36	20.0	13	481	8.2	29.1	2.0	34.3	21.2
301	Guisborough	Langbaurgh	107	63	2.7	146	13.9	35	258	14.2	48.7	3.0	56.1	30.4
302	Arthuret	Carlisle	129	33	2.5	60	11.8	19	255	10.5	36.8	4.5	68.7	37.0
303	Teesville	Langbaurgh	131	76	2.1	115	13.1	26	351	14.3	36.7	3.2	33.2	22.8
304	Tanfield	Derwentside	107	32	2.6	84	14.3	29	303	16.4	44.3	2.8	42.1	21.6
305	Ingleton	Teesdale	89	5	2.2	11	18.2	2	506	7.9	19.9	1.4	50.7	37.5
306	Stamfordham	Castle Morpeth	140	14	0.8	8	17.1	12	519	2.0	18.3	3.3	67.4	25.7

307	Sleekburn	Wansbeck	123	42	2.5	75	12.5	13	290	10.1	52.3	2.2	67.9	28.0
308	Bedlington West	Wansbeck	119	44	2.6	87	12.6	16	323	9.2	42.4	3.1	58.8	17.8
309	Easington Village	Easington	117	19	2.6	47	12.7	7	438	6.5	42.1	2.3	39.7	2.6
310	West Park	South Tyneside	112	74	1.9	120	16.3	36	386	10.0	45.2	2.4	35.3	19.9
311	Newtorn	Copeland	116	29	2.5	65	13.3	20	360	10.1	49.9	2.8	32.1	37.3
312	Wolsingham	Wear Valley	111	31	2.5	66	14.0	12	388	8.2	38.1	2.7	47.5	17.5
313	Harrowgate Hill	Darlington	131	55	1.5	62	15.1	28	446	8.9	42.8	2.9	15.2	25.4
314	Shafto	Sedgefield	110	27	2.7	63	13.1	19	248	12.9	48.4	1.8	81.6	27.7
315	Penrith North	Eden	120	33	1.2	35	17.8	24	480	6.5	34.6	2.5	29.4	20.2
316	Denton	Newcastle upon Tyne	118	130	2.5	234	12.8	33	240	10.3	52.4	3.1	68.1	22.9
317	Waver	Allerdale	82	13	2.1	31	19.0	16	471	6.6	19.6	3.1	43.0	18.2
318	Newham	Middlesbrough	121	72	2.0	115	14.4	61	490	10.5	23.1	2.0	28.6	12.5
319	Boltons	Allerdale	90	14	2.0	28	18.4	14	504	7.4	20.0	2.9	29.1	36.6
320	Whessoe	Darlington	11	25	1.2	21	16.2	12	591	6.2	15.1	2.0	25.2	22.6
321	Washington West	Sunderland	107	82	2.0	178	16.1	116	281	13.7	39.9	3.0	63.4	23.3
322	Pelton	Chester-le-Street	76	29	3.4	133	14.5	36	205	14.6	51.6	4.0	59.3	27.1
323	Stainsby	Stockton-on-Tees	103	45	2.6	125	14.1	43	259	17.8	45.4	4.6	67.4	29.1
324	Coniston	South Lakeland	91	9	1.9	18	18.5	5	493	4.9	28.1	1.0	53.0	13.3
325	Langbaurgh	Langbaurgh	120	69	2.3	130	13.1	46	277	17.5	47.5	2.8	46.2	37.1
326	Stainton and Thornton	Middlesbrough	84	29	2.4	89	17.4	41	145	21.1	43.1	4.6	67.4	35.3
327	Currock	Carlisle	118	55	2.2	103	13.7	38	365	9.5	51.6	1.9	44.5	27.8
328	Chowdene	Gateshead	115	97	2.3	183	13.6	33	250	10.0	49.2	3.7	63.1	20.8
329	Hemlington	Middlesbrough	114	34	2.4	82	13.4	41	147	19.2	43.6	4.4	71.6	21.7
330	Fens	Hartlepool	134	73	1.5	82	14.3	42	334	14.2	33.8	4.4	32.4	27.1
331	Kells	Copeland	98	22	2.0	42	17.1	14	343	7.4	49.9	2.9	51.6	33.9
332	Acomb with Sandhoe	Tynedale	133	18	1.9	24	12.8	6	434	6.0	32.4	2.7	50.6	28.6
333	Brough	Eden	103	9	1.8	16	17.1	7	466	7.0	21.1	2.8	43.6	27.6
334	Park	Middlesbrough	104	42	2.6	100	13.7	27	346	15.4	47.0	2.9	22.7	25.7
335	Pelaw & Heworth	Gateshead	102	89	2.8	211	13.1	38	139	13.1	58.7	4.4	72.9	21.3
336	Newbiggin West	Wansbeck	108	31	2.7	74	12.7	16	278	10.4	51.1	3.2	57.9	28.4
337	Northside	Allerdale	75	12	3.0	55	15.9	10	54	22.6	61.3	4.5	89.7	54.8
338	Denton Holme	Carlisle	123	54	1.6	71	15.1	36	330	10.0	54.8	2.7	40.8	27.5
339	Crawcrook and Greenside	Gateshead	109	75	2.6	176	12.0	50	380	8.8	47.2	3.1	30.8	20.1
340	Pegswood	Castle Morpeth	131	33	2.6	66	10.0	13	106	7.4	46.9	5.5	79.1	28.9
341	Whitburn and Marsden	South Tyneside	113	74	2.8	161	11.5	22	192	13.7	53.5	3.1	73.4	24.4

342	Skelton	Langbaurgh	128	66	2.6	133	10.4	29	287	16.6	41.7	3.9	40.9	35.5
343	Hunwick	Wear Valley	131	17	2.9	33	8.7	8	340	11.1	36.3	5.5	27.5	33.3
344	Longhoughton	Alnwick	97	9	1.0	10	20.9	23	372	4.9	27.5	2.6	89.4	16.7
345	Morton	Carlisle	93	47	2.5	109	15.3	9	142	7.5	55.8	6.3	82.4	28.1
346	Romaldkirk	Teesdale	74	5	3.2	21	15.0	3	550	4.4	24.8	1.9	41.6	6.7
347	Howletch	Easington	126	31	2.2	66	12.1	27	221	11.6	35.7	3.7	84.8	18.1
348	Walney North	Barrow-in-Furness	133	54	1.6	59	13.5	26	364	8.5	41.8	3.1	44.5	22.9
349	Barnard Castle East	Teesdale	66	13	2.1	39	20.3	14	321	7.4	47.6	3.2	60.2	29.5
350	Wingrove	Newcastle upon Tyne	100	80	2.0	157	16.1	58	267	11.4	53.4	4.2	42.4	22.2
351	Haltwhistle	Tynedale	125	37	2.1	59	12.4	17	366	5.8	48.4	3.1	50.3	37.5
352	Prudhoe South	Tynedale	131	29	2.7	59	9.0	10	332	7.8	40.9	4.9	43.5	20.0
353	Ouston	Chester-le-Street	109	24	1.6	37	16.4	30	530	7.8	22.8	1.8	30.2	15.4
354	Lemington	Newcastle upon Tyne	110	82	2.1	159	14.2	53	268	13.5	46.5	4.1	45.2	20.2
355	Park	Hartlepool	89	48	2.2	111	16.5	21	187	16.3	44.6	4.4	64.5	27.1
356	Brampton	Carlisle	114	34	1.8	52	14.8	17	377	10.0	35.5	1.6	65.2	19.7
357	Seaham	Easington	102	33	2.6	82	13.2	12	252	8.7	54.0	3.7	62.2	24.4
358	Whickham North	Gateshead	93	81	3.1	256	12.3	44	310	10.5	47.5	3.4	47.5	17.6
359	Whinfell	South Lakeland	118	10	1.0	9	17.5	7	648	4.0	8.3	1.6	28.0	13.8
360	Chester Central	Chester-le-Street	111	12	1.9	25	14.7	17	441	8.9	49.2	2.5	14.2	21.3
361	Haughton East	Darlington	112	58	2.2	115	13.2	45	376	9.6	40.2	2.4	47.9	20.4
362	Hensingham	Copeland	105	35	2.6	83	12.4	21	228	10.3	50.2	2.8	78.8	30.1
363	Elvet	Durham	95	16	2.1	37	15.9	10	362	6.1	56.6	1.4	65.8	24.5
364	Haverigg	Copeland	83	7	3.2	24	12.9	4	436	7.9	46.5	1.7	36.6	27.8
365	Frizington	Copeland	126	25	2.5	49	10.1	11	176	16.1	46.8	5.4	57.4	30.4
366	Bankside	Langbaurgh	91	31	2.4	85	15.0	39	174	18.6	55.4	3.1	63.1	38.0
367	Bishop Auckland Town	Wear Valley	120	38	2.5	75	10.8	14	353	11.8	49.3	3.3	23.4	25.8
368	Appleby Bongate	Eden	127	10	1.6	13	13.5	13	511	3.8	26.1	3.3	39.0	32.1
369	Norton	Stockton-on-Tees	99	48	1.8	93	16.3	41	450	11.5	42.3	1.6	23.1	26.3
370	Hawkshead	South Lakeland	104	11	1.3	12	17.6	6	497	5.4	16.9	2.3	56.5	20.7
371	Saltburn	Langbaurgh	111	58	2.2	105	12.9	19	402	14.8	38.4	1.9	30.2	14.5
372	Urpeth	Chester-le-Street	120	19	1.9	39	12.9	19	494	9.0	26.6	2.5	21.8	10.8
373	Guide Post	Wansbeck	81	28	2.2	69	16.8	19	430	7.4	38.7	1.9	48.0	26.5
374	Distington	Copeland	97	22	1.6	34	17.2	22	262	12.3	39.6	4.2	58.7	30.6
375	Etherley	Teesdale	79	11	2.4	43	16.4	9	379	13.6	34.7	2.7	34.5	21.4
376	Low Furness	South Lakeland	106	25	1.3	26	17.1	12	622	4.8	15.0	1.9	21.5	9.4

			1	2	3	4	5	6	7	8	9	10	11	12
377	Weetslade	North Tyneside	107	92	1.8	143	14.9	47	464	6.7	37.9	1.9	38.2	15.2
378	South	Easington	87	11	3.2	42	11.8	9	180	13.2	59.4	4.3	58.4	35.7
379	Benton	North Tyneside	89	79	2.6	197	14.0	32	312	11.9	49.2	2.6	49.9	21.4
380	Penrith South	Eden	90	18	1.7	31	17.5	11	417	6.5	35.9	3.1	46.2	24.6
381	Ennerdale	Copeland	94	13	1.7	24	17.0	15	495	8.0	22.2	2.9	26.5	21.4
382	Pennington	South Lakeland	113	16	1.6	19	14.8	4	534	3.9	24.6	3.1	33.5	17.6
383	Newburn	Newcastle upon Tyne	94	73	2.6	199	13.1	49	201	13.7	55.9	3.2	67.0	26.1
384	Pallion	Sunderland	96	95	2.3	214	14.1	45	291	14.9	49.0	3.7	36.5	20.8
385	Dawdon	Easington	79	42	2.8	142	14.3	43	105	11.6	61.8	6.8	70.6	25.9
386	Howgate	Copeland	82	20	2.0	46	17.1	22	304	9.7	41.8	3.2	61.9	29.6
387	Hartside	Eden	99	9	2.3	18	13.6	6	606	5.7	15.0	1.1	40.2	30.4
388	Simpasture	Sedgefield	105	22	2.3	39	12.9	9	170	14.3	51.3	3.3	78.9	36.7
389	St Peter's	Sunderland	102	83	2.3	188	13.1	52	289	14.5	54.9	3.1	37.7	16.8
390	Harraby	Carlisle	99	54	2.0	96	14.8	27	275	9.1	43.7	4.6	58.8	23.7
391	Seatonville	North Tyneside	90	76	2.2	168	15.2	35	410	9.6	41.0	2.0	41.6	11.7
392	Elm Tree	Stockton-on-Tees	132	35	1.3	35	13.2	24	515	11.1	23.5	1.5	27.0	11.5
393	Murton West	Easington	92	30	4.1	113	7.1	6	195	8.7	61.9	3.6	74.4	23.0
394	Alnwick Hotspur	Alnwick	116	20	2.4	40	10.8	7	392	6.2	49.5	2.1	51.2	15.9
395	Dearham	Allerdale	93	15	1.8	27	16.2	13	425	9.1	35.7	2.5	35.1	20.5
396	Spennymoor	Sedgefield	118	50	2.0	92	11.9	38	455	9.0	35.9	2.2	29.1	24.5
397	Blackhill	Derwentside	121	43	2.3	81	10.2	17	164	29.0	49.3	3.7	49.5	26.7
398	Bedlington East	Wansbeck	81	30	2.5	85	14.8	25	315	9.4	51.0	2.5	58.1	30.1
399	Penrith East	Eden	107	35	1.9	61	13.7	16	399	7.3	41.7	1.7	59.0	14.9
400	Framwelgate	Durham	102	38	2.1	74	13.5	19	440	6.0	35.5	2.5	47.8	21.4
401	Lowther	Eden	130	13	0.7	7	15.4	8	567	5.0	15.4	1.5	50.0	11.8
402	Ponteland North	Castle Morpeth	105	17	2.9	38	10.5	4	420	5.9	32.3	2.0	69.1	21.1
403	Heaton	Newcastle upon Tyne	105	85	1.9	162	13.7	50	288	11.0	58.6	2.9	47.4	18.1
404	Chollerton with Whittingtn	Tynedale	89	8	2.0	17	15.4	8	397	4.9	23.1	4.1	66.4	23.5
405	Marsh House	Stockton-on-Tees	100	45	1.3	69	16.7	65	472	10.6	24.3	2.4	27.4	21.2
406	Hartford and West	Blyth Valley	109	30	2.0	65	12.7	32	212	14.5	42.6	3.2	76.5	37.3
407	Gilesgate	Tynedale	62	6	1.8	16	19.6	10	347	7.4	47.0	3.6	42.8	28.1
408	Crummock	Allerdale	95	11	1.7	16	15.6	5	565	6.5	14.6	1.9	34.4	3.7
409	Grange	Hartlepool	119	58	1.3	63	14.1	36	560	11.0	31.5	1.0	12.1	20.4
410	St. John's	Allerdale	93	34	1.3	48	17.4	29	542	8.6	39.3	1.5	8.2	15.7
411	Dene	Newcastle upon Tyne	107	124	2.0	194	12.7	37	444	7.2	45.8	1.8	37.9	10.9

No.	Ward	District												
412	Linthorpe	Middlesbrough	110	42	1.6	66	13.8	35	403	14.3	43.4	2.6	14.2	16.7
413	Kendal Far Cross	South Lakeland	127	23	1.9	31	10.3	6	342	6.8	47.0	2.5	64.2	26.0
414	Middleton in Teesdale	Teesdale	91	12	2.1	26	14.3	7	395	8.8	34.2	2.1	56.4	23.7
415	Cockton Hill	Wear Valley	71	30	2.0	80	17.3	26	558	6.8	35.9	1.6	12.8	13.5
416	Egremont South	Copeland	132	37	1.6	41	10.9	12	339	8.0	38.0	2.9	64.9	34.6
417	Burnopfield	Derwentside	99	37	2.7	98	10.8	17	371	11.3	41.6	2.2	44.6	19.1
418	Redcar	Langbaurgh	122	50	2.4	96	8.8	16	424	13.5	45.2	1.8	18.7	31.7
419	Sedgefield	Sedgefield	90	34	1.7	66	15.9	29	548	7.1	24.8	1.3	35.4	15.0
420	Haughton West	Darlington	107	35	1.8	59	13.2	20	359	9.5	40.5	3.2	41.7	30.3
421	Morpeth Stobhill	Castle Morpeth	102	30	3.0	74	9.0	7	404	7.1	39.1	2.7	46.4	20.0
422	Moorclose	Allerdale	88	31	1.7	57	16.2	21	131	14.0	48.7	4.5	84.9	41.4
423	Valley	North Tyneside	86	68	2.7	193	12.3	41	231	12.6	53.8	2.9	63.7	22.4
424	Bank Top	Darlington	85	23	2.1	56	14.7	23	373	10.5	49.7	3.9	14.7	20.9
425	Waldridge	Chester-le-Street	90	9	1.6	21	16.0	17	649	6.4	16.0	1.3	4.2	12.3
426	North Shields	North Tyneside	98	77	1.8	144	14.2	45	355	10.7	52.7	2.0	39.5	18.7
427	Mickley	Tynedale	85	10	1.9	26	15.5	11	617	4.9	25.8	1.7	12.7	14.0
428	Seaton Moor	Allerdale	88	39	1.6	67	16.2	31	447	9.1	29.7	2.4	37.7	23.4
429	Alnwick Castle	Alnwick	88	20	2.1	43	14.1	12	327	7.1	45.7	2.8	65.7	26.5
430	Elizabeth	Berwick-upon-Tweed	121	24	1.1	23	13.8	9	468	5.5	41.1	1.8	42.3	14.3
431	Colton & Haverthwaite	South Lakeland	108	15	2.4	31	10.3	4	513	5.8	22.2	2.0	45.5	13.9
432	Tynemouth	North Tyneside	102	80	2.0	151	12.7	38	325	10.9	49.4	2.9	43.3	16.7
433	Washington East	Sunderland	99	89	1.9	200	13.5	112	297	12.8	37.9	3.3	57.8	17.7
434	Consett North	Derwentside	88	24	3.0	72	10.4	10	257	25.6	49.2	2.9	32.0	21.5
435	Seghill	Blyth Valley	89	19	2.5	45	12.3	9	279	11.1	49.6	2.0	74.2	38.8
436	Prudhoe West	Tynedale	91	14	2.2	37	13.3	13	469	5.9	35.3	2.8	31.6	9.8
437	Croxdale	Durham	93	10	2.3	23	12.5	5	293	10.2	35.1	5.3	53.8	22.9
438	Milnthorpe	South Lakeland	107	21	1.9	36	12.3	10	544	4.0	29.5	1.5	48.6	18.3
439	Gilesgate Moor	Durham	97	22	1.9	45	13.5	15	522	6.9	29.3	1.9	28.5	15.9
440	Chester North	Chester-le-Street	111	37	2.7	89	8.4	10	348	10.0	42.4	2.5	50.2	15.8
441	Haydon	Tynedale	97	15	2.0	33	13.0	9	305	9.3	34.5	4.8	56.3	23.8
442	Lesbury	Alnwick	110	17	2.2	31	10.4	5	459	6.7	29.1	1.7	56.1	37.8
443	Washington South	Sunderland	98	69	2.0	165	12.8	115	318	12.4	33.9	2.4	68.8	18.4
444	Carville	Durham	107	29	2.1	54	11.1	11	477	6.7	32.1	2.5	32.7	25.0
445	Lanchester	Derwentside	120	47	1.9	70	10.2	14	467	11.3	28.4	1.7	32.2	13.3
446	Dalton North	Barrow-in-Furness	118	51	1.6	67	11.7	26	526	7.6	36.1	1.9	13.5	20.5

			1	2	3	4	5	6	7	8	9	10	11
447	Benfieldside	Derwentshire	111	45	1.8	74	11.8	24	400	19.2	36.6	1.5	29.3	19.8
448	Broomhaugh and Riding	Tynedale	116	8	1.2	8	13.5	5	636	4.5	24.5	1.3	15.8	0.0
449	Craster and Rennington	Alnwick	123	7	1.7	9	10.5	2	387	6.3	25.5	3.2	68.1	63.6
450	Islandshire	Berwick-upon-Tweed	106	18	1.7	29	12.7	14	393	7.2	30.4	2.9	58.2	19.7
451	Parkside	Barrow-in-Furness	113	49	1.4	62	12.9	23	533	8.1	38.8	1.5	12.6	13.2
452	Pierremont	Darlington	98	44	1.1	52	16.2	31	551	7.2	42.7	1.0	17.6	9.5
453	Westoe	South Tyneside	101	58	1.4	84	14.6	44	389	9.0	49.4	2.6	29.9	17.0
454	Streatlam and Whorlton	Teesdale	74	5	2.7	17	12.9	4	384	10.6	25.9	2.0	65.4	20.0
455	Ulgham	Castle Morpeth	78	17	2.2	48	14.3	17	319	9.0	39.9	3.8	56.0	21.0
456	Ellen	Allerdale	106	18	2.3	34	10.2	6	379	8.6	26.6	2.3	31.8	13.3
457	Kader	Middlesbrough	88	50	1.4	75	16.1	25	601	8.5	21.7	1.5	8.9	15.7
458	St Michael's	Sunderland	92	87	1.9	171	13.5	40	505	9.3	31.1	1.7	24.1	10.9
459	Fellgate and Hedworth	South Tyneside	104	71	2.2	156	10.7	41	133	17.2	49.1	5.9	63.0	25.7
460	Gilesgate	Durham	77	29	2.6	83	12.6	17	260	9.0	52.9	2.9	69.7	24.2
461	Yewdale	Carlisle	87	40	1.4	71	16.0	55	426	6.7	31.5	3.2	43.3	13.6
462	Newsham and New Delaval	Blyth Valley	102	32	1.9	70	12.0	28	352	10.9	41.0	2.5	48.0	16.8
463	Seaton	Wansbeck	97	32	2.1	77	11.8	24	344	8.1	41.7	2.8	59.3	19.2
464	Whitley Bay	North Tyneside	111	75	2.1	144	9.9	31	412	12.6	51.4	1.5	30.2	14.4
465	Priestpopple	Tynedale	96	24	2.8	68	9.1	10	271	9.3	48.6	4.1	56.6	35.4
466	Shilbottle	Alnwick	98	23	1.8	40	12.3	9	261	9.6	41.7	3.6	72.4	16.7
467	Kendal Nether	South Lakeland	79	14	2.1	37	14.0	8	488	5.2	47.6	1.0	46.6	31.3
468	Whitton	Stockton-on-Tees	109	20	2.0	37	10.4	13	435	9.7	30.0	2.4	38.7	24.6
469	Ellington	Castle Morpeth	112	22	2.4	48	8.3	12	531	3.8	22.8	3.4	34.3	12.7
470	Irthing	Carlisle	93	14	1.4	19	14.8	8	462	8.1	15.1	3.7	37.4	10.0
471	Sedbergh	South Lakeland	80	20	1.8	42	14.9	13	473	5.7	30.8	2.1	47.9	16.9
472	Kendal Glebelands	South Lakeland	85	12	1.3	19	16.4	9	306	10.1	44.1	4.1	46.8	27.3
473	College	Darlington	99	26	1.3	33	14.4	13	540	9.1	33.3	1.2	20.4	9.2
474	Stakeford	Wansbeck	96	26	1.5	40	13.9	11	509	6.5	34.2	1.6	34.7	13.0
475	Dormanstown	Langbaurgh	93	58	2.5	137	10.3	27	203	17.7	51.0	4.2	50.9	26.5
476	Roosecote	Barrow-in-Furness	94	38	1.9	74	12.5	26	517	8.0	28.0	2.5	17.2	17.8
477	Greystoke	Eden	119	13	0.9	9	13.2	5	579	5.7	20.8	1.3	39.0	22.6
478	Ford	Berwick-upon-Tweed	93	9	2.0	19	12.1	4	374	6.2	27.7	3.2	71.1	57.6
479	Cullercoats	North Tyneside	104	108	2.0	171	10.6	21	501	7.1	39.5	1.4	30.7	16.3
480	Kendal Strickland	South Lakeland	106	17	2.3	32	9.1	5	453	6.5	40.4	2.1	38.2	14.3
481	Gainford & Winston	Teesdale	68	10	1.4	19	17.7	11	576	6.2	20.5	1.3	35.7	17.9

482 Jesmond	Newcastle upon Tyne	107	68	1.4	115	12.7	41	357	10.9	47.9	1.6	51.1	11.3
483 Dalton South	Barrow-in-Furness	108	46	1.6	66	11.7	24	429	8.3	36.7	2.9	31.2	20.7
484 Belah	Carlisle	113	54	1.5	71	11.3	21	535	6.1	31.1	1.4	35.5	11.5
485 Wampool	Allerdale	118	22	1.1	21	12.3	8	541	5.4	13.8	3.7	27.6	26.7
486 Allendale	Tynedale	99	15	2.2	32	10.3	6	485	8.9	28.7	1.6	37.7	12.2
487 Low Fell	Gateshead	104	79	1.5	113	12.5	41	527	6.2	41.2	1.6	19.5	9.5
488 Central	Blyth Valley	90	28	1.6	53	13.9	24	439	9.7	50.1	1.3	31.7	17.5
489 Throston	Hartlepool	80	27	2.1	71	13.0	18	247	14.9	48.1	3.2	55.5	27.1
490 Village	Blyth Valley	115	37	1.1	42	12.4	21	521	7.3	28.4	1.8	29.6	11.2
491 Park	Easington	75	13	1.8	31	14.7	10	375	7.0	42.1	3.4	45.2	26.3
492 Elwick	Hartlepool	105	14	1.0	13	14.0	6	603	6.5	14.1	1.6	27.3	0.0
493 Kirkby Stephen	Eden	95	16	2.0	33	11.3	7	449	7.1	29.7	2.3	47.3	21.7
494 Yarm	Stockton-on-Tees	97	39	1.3	61	13.9	47	635	5.7	16.0	1.1	23.4	12.4
495 Dacre	Eden	81	8	1.7	14	14.3	2	596	4.4	17.4	1.5	41.4	28.6
496 Marsh	Allerdale	123	19	1.7	27	8.6	7	608	5.1	15.9	1.9	26.4	21.3
497 All Saints	Allerdale	99	31	2.1	60	10.2	12	385	9.5	34.6	2.4	52.0	11.6
498 Arnside	South Lakeland	89	14	1.6	26	13.3	5	598	7.4	26.0	1.0	21.0	5.7
499 Northamshire	Berwick-upon-Tweed	94	12	0.9	11	15.6	10	432	3.8	30.4	3.5	60.8	23.7
500 Bournmoor	Chester-le-Street	109	27	2.1	52	8.8	6	474	7.9	30.6	2.0	36.8	14.3
501 North Sunderland	Berwick-upon-Tweed	93	13	2.2	30	10.5	4	428	10.1	38.7	1.4	45.3	19.4
502 Hart	Hartlepool	105	27	1.1	29	13.3	23	514	10.5	23.2	1.5	29.9	28.0
503 Warcop	Eden	105	10	1.6	14	11.1	5	556	4.1	15.1	2.9	38.7	21.4
504 East Tynedale	Tynedale	109	10	1.4	13	11.4	5	419	6.1	25.1	3.3	59.2	25.7
505 Walney South	Barrow-in-Furness	121	61	1.3	61	10.1	22	460	7.2	42.8	2.4	23.5	18.4
506 Ormesby	Langbaurgh	83	27	1.4	43	15.2	17	587	9.0	21.7	1.3	16.6	21.0
507 Levens	South Lakeland	75	11	1.4	19	15.8	6	662	3.4	13.7	0.6	30.4	17.5
508 Hartburn	Castle Morpeth	125	10	0.8	6	11.4	4	478	3.4	12.0	3.0	76.3	34.8
509 Westerhope	Newcastle upon Tyne	93	96	1.5	146	12.8	51	507	6.7	31.4	2.3	26.0	10.3
510 Egremont North	Copeland	111	38	1.5	51	10.4	25	269	9.9	38.2	4.4	65.4	33.3
511 Lazonby	Eden	84	7	1.4	11	14.3	5	566	6.3	18.3	1.1	46.5	8.7
512 Morpeth Central	Castle Morpeth	75	12	1.4	34	12.7	9	367	7.6	52.6	2.2	46.9	23.1
513 Bishop Middleham	Sedgefield	90	9	2.1	23	9.8	5	458	6.9	33.2	1.9	46.8	25.7
514 Longbeck	Langbaurgh	90	48	1.3	79	13.9	39	580	8.8	19.7	2.0	7.7	23.4
515 Wigton	Allerdale	90	33	2.1	75	10.5	15	311	9.1	43.4	3.7	55.2	35.0
516 Stanhope	Wear Valley	107	23	2.2	45	7.8	6	431	9.3	36.8	2.0	47.3	32.8

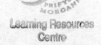

ID	Ward	District											
517	Bransty	Copeland	92	25	1.7	48	11.8	18	454	8.2	36.6	2.1	33.9	22.0
518	Eamont	Eden	95	9	1.7	14	11.4	4	594	7.0	20.2	0.8	38.0	19.2
519	Shap	Eden	82	8	1.7	17	13.2	5	382	8.8	29.2	3.5	48.9	42.3
520	Castleside	Derwentside	72	10	1.8	22	14.0	6	406	18.4	28.8	2.0	31.1	12.8
521	Wensleydale	Blyth Valley	106	37	1.1	46	12.4	43	618	5.1	23.8	1.6	15.7	12.4
522	Bishopsgrath	Stockton-on-Tees	96	46	1.1	64	13.6	61	599	8.6	18.8	1.5	12.6	12.4
523	Rift House	Hartlepool	93	41	1.7	75	11.7	27	510	10.2	36.3	1.8	9.7	26.9
524	Mowden	Darlington	116	40	1.0	32	11.4	8	674	4.0	20.4	0.1	7.0	6.5
525	Hartburn	Stockton-on-Tees	101	52	1.2	70	12.6	38	660	6.9	13.8	0.9	3.1	11.6
526	Orton with Tebay	Eden	94	8	1.5	13	13.2	5	500	5.6	24.2	3.0	34.1	6.9
527	St. Bridget's	Allerdale	87	12	1.2	16	14.3	8	561	7.4	18.1	1.6	31.4	15.9
528	Normanby	Langbaurgh	106	42	1.8	67	9.3	14	487	10.4	25.4	2.8	16.1	20.3
529	Byerley	Sedgefield	98	28	1.7	44	10.8	11	309	9.9	55.6	3.9	34.3	26.7
530	Bootle	Copeland	71	9	1.7	20	14.3	7	609	3.3	18.2	1.6	44.3	27.8
531	Newton Hall	Durham	131	44	0.6	26	10.7	26	675	3.1	11.2	0.5	6.2	11.6
532	Seaton Delaval	Blyth Valley	56	16	2.0	58	15.0	20	416	9.2	42.1	1.7	45.6	12.5
533	Fairfield	Stockton-on-Tees	96	46	1.7	70	15.0	14	582	7.9	22.9	1.4	18.9	15.2
534	Kendal Heron Hill	South Lakeland	91	15	0.8	13	15.2	15	664	3.4	18.0	1.3	6.2	11.1
535	Lakes Ambleside	South Lakeland	81	20	1.5	35	13.6	12	491	5.0	32.4	1.8	48.8	16.2
536	Stanwix Urban	Carlisle	103	45	1.3	54	11.4	20	492	9.0	37.2	1.4	27.3	11.9
537	Howden	Wear Valley	88	16	2.6	44	8.1	6	336	15.3	35.7	3.5	35.9	40.5
538	Wolviston	Stockton-on-Tees	87	8	0.7	8	15.9	11	626	7.3	18.1	1.1	14.6	12.2
539	Heighington	Darlington	83	12	1.3	18	14.0	6	646	5.1	18.5	1.1	17.7	15.9
540	Cartmel	South Lakeland	82	13	1.6	23	12.9	4	614	6.6	29.0	0.7	22.3	22.6
541	Windermere Bowness	South Lakeland	95	13	1.2	15	12.8	8	465	7.5	28.8	2.1	42.0	13.6
542	Great Corby and Geltsdale	Carlisle	82	11	1.0	13	15.3	9	623	6.4	13.8	1.1	28.3	10.6
543	Barnard Castle West	Teesdale	91	18	1.6	31	11.6	8	463	5.5	39.3	2.2	40.2	21.4
544	Hartley	Blyth Valley	87	36	2.0	82	10.5	20	452	9.5	32.5	2.1	33.7	22.0
545	Warkworth	Alnwick	77	12	1.7	26	13.0	14	525	5.9	26.0	1.7	40.2	17.6
546	Kirby	Middlesbrough	108	48	1.5	65	9.6	16	645	8.8	22.8	0.6	5.3	12.1
547	Stainburn	Allerdale	137	25	1.4	25	6.0	5	557	8.9	29.1	1.1	22.1	21.1
548	St Germain's	Langbaurgh	101	44	2.2	93	7.4	8	427	11.7	31.4	1.9	39.5	20.9
549	Kendal Castle	South Lakeland	112	18	1.3	22	9.5	6	578	3.5	26.5	1.7	40.1	11.1
550	Hillcrest	Copeland	105	21	0.8	20	12.4	19	656	3.8	19.1	0.8	21.9	16.0
551	Askham	Eden	103	8	1.2	9	11.1	2	613	2.3	17.5	1.7	51.6	21.1

657	Lakes Grasmere	South Lakeland	96	11	0.5	5	6.2	3	523	6.3	23.0	49.3	0.0
658	Morpeth Kirkhill	Castle Morpeth	44	11	0.9	20	10.9	7	538	4.5	26.8	40.7	15.6
659	Tofthill & Lands	Teesdale	125	6	0.9	4	0.0	0	545	6.8	17.2	13.6	23.5
660	Hedgeley	Alnwick	43	3	0.9	6	10.3	3	364	5.9	17.1	77.3	42.9
661	Broughton	South Lakeland	67	12	1.5	26	4.8	4	595	5.1	15.4	28.4	12.1
662	Neville's Cross	Durham	49	16	1.3	43	7.6	10	654	4.8	30.1	14.1	11.8
663	Dalton	Allerdale	29	4	1.1	14	11.1	6	532	7.6	17.5	32.5	13.9
664	Beadnell	Berwick-upon-Tweed	49	4	2.3	17	3.2	1	370	8.2	25.7	59.8	14.3
665	Greta	Teesdale	41	2	1.9	9	5.9	1	457	7.8	14.5	53.3	20.0
666	Leazes	Tynedale	62	12	1.4	25	4.9	3	665	2.9	27.9	15.8	8.5
667	Hummersknott	Darlington	44	15	1.2	35	7.5	5	672	2.9	15.4	7.6	1.1
668	Hutton	South Lakeland	40	4	0.7	7	10.0	4	616	3.8	6.4	37.6	6.1
669	Upper North Tyne	Tynedale	70	5	1.2	7	3.7	1	414	6.0	22.2	75.6	35.0
670	Cartmel Fell	South Lakeland	40	5	1.0	12	8.3	2	619	6.8	13.6	30.7	21.2
671	Crosby Ravensworth	Eden	55	6	1.1	8	5.4	2	625	2.7	11.1	44.7	13.0
672	Appleby	Eden	64	6	1.1	11	3.6	1	555	3.9	33.4	46.0	32.3
673	Shincliffe	Durham	74	8	0.9	10	1.8	1	673	3.2	15.2	17.3	2.5
674	Hutton	Langbaurgh	41	11	0.6	18	7.1	9	676	4.6	5.7	6.4	4.7
675	Heddon-on-the-Wall	Castle Morpeth	61	11	1.3	18	0.0	0	653	4.6	17.7	27.2	7.9
676	Wanney	Tynedale	43	3	1.7	11	0.0	0	476	3.8	25.6	50.9	27.8
677	Hamsterley & South Bedburn	Teesdale	38	2	1.8	8	0.0	0	516	8.2	19.7	36.6	27.3
678	Harbottle	Alnwick	38	2	0.8	4	3.6	1	537	5.4	13.9	64.1	50.0

622	Beckermet	Copeland	83	21	0.9	21	9.6	10	489	6.1	22.4	2.5	43.6	24.3
623	Wylam	Tynedale	64	11	1.1	18	11.3	6	624	4.4	26.7	1.3	21.6	5.7
624	Cornerstone with Lartingtn	Teesdale	36	2	3.6	18	4.8	1	569	3.6	22.7	2.9	29.3	20.0
625	Hencotes	Tynedale	79	20	2.1	47	4.9	3	423	6.2	42.4	2.0	51.7	25.0
626	Glebe	Stockton-on-Tees	83	31	1.0	41	8.9	20	655	6.7	17.0	0.7	7.1	12.3
627	Tipalt	Tynedale	27	2	2.0	14	12.0	3	442	8.3	28.9	3.5	37.5	28.6
628	Wooler	Tynedale	56	10	1.4	23	10.5	4	361	6.0	38.9	1.9	57.7	23.4
629	Startforth East	Berwick-upon-Tweed	43	2	1.7	8	11.1	3	486	8.4	18.4	1.2	47.6	25.0
630	Harrington	Allerdale	55	11	0.7	15	13.5	13	642	6.0	20.9	0.8	8.5	20.6
531	Bellingham	Tynedale	71	6	1.2	11	9.4	3	326	6.0	39.2	3.9	68.3	12.5
632	Meltwhaite	Copeland	50	6	0.8	9	13.6	6	575	5.0	15.6	1.6	44.1	8.3
633	Ravenstonedale	Eden	45	3	1.7	11	10.7	3	536	4.9	14.1	2.5	46.3	10.5
634	West Tynedale	Tynedale	49	4	2.3	16	7.7	3	369	11.4	20.8	3.1	59.0	31.8
635	Seascale	Copeland	94	16	1.7	16	7.0	5	643	3.5	16.0	0.8	49.6	10.8
636	Windermere Applethwaite	South Lakeland	65	7	1.7	17	7.7	2	604	4.6	23.4	0.8	45.8	6.7
637	Park West	Darlington	72	20	1.1	30	9.2	7	627	6.1	31.3	0.5	21.3	9.3
638	Skelton	Eden	79	8	1.1	8	9.3	4	637	5.3	39.5	0.9	39.5	9.3
639	Crake Valley	South Lakeland	88	11	0.9	11	7.7	3	610	6.6	22.4	0.7	34.3	17.1
640	Morpeth North	Castle Morpeth	95	22	0.5	11	8.3	8	659	5.1	17.6	0.7	15.4	4.9
641	Redesdale	Tynedale	53	4	1.3	9	10.7	8	499	3.1	29.4	1.3	78.1	11.7
642	Marton	Middlesbrough	91	29	0.6	23	8.5	19	641	7.1	13.1	1.5	11.7	4.7
643	St Mary's	North Tyneside	69	49	1.0	65	9.8	21	669	5.2	18.4	0.2	6.3	2.9
644	Grange	South Lakeland	83	22	1.4	37	6.1	4	639	5.7	33.7	0.3	23.1	14.3
645	Endmoor	South Lakeland	49	9	0.9	16	12.3		631	3.6	14.8	2.2	22.2	5.5
646	Belmont	Durham	73	17	0.6	15	10.1	15	670	3.5	9.1	1.0	5.9	8.3
647	Hebron, Hepscott & Mitford	Castle Morpeth	130	16	1.2	13	0.0	0	612	4.8	13.9	1.5	36.7	11.8
648	Chatton	Berwick-upon-Tweed	51	3	1.3	7	10.0	2	391	4.8	19.8	3.1	85.6	36.8
649	Lyne	Carlisle	45	8	2.1	34	7.4		570	5.0	9.2	3.0	33.6	9.3
650	Parkside	Blyth Valley	64	19	0.6	27	10.8	69	584	8.4	18.1	1.5	20.3	13.4
651	Hayton	Carlisle	57	10	1.7	28	7.3	6	577	5.3	15.1	2.4	28.5	9.7
652	Ulverston North	South Lakeland	66	10	1.3	19	7.5	3	568	6.0	38.6	1.3	24.0	20.5
653	Windermere Bowness	South Lakeland	52	9	1.3	14	10.9	5	585	6.0	30.6	0.8	30.1	16.3
654	Burton & Holme	South Lakeland	46	8	1.5	25	9.3	5	644	4.3	19.3	2.1	21.5	11.1
655	Ponteland East	Castle Morpeth	90	20	1.2	25	4.3	2	652	4.1	16.2	1.2	19.1	13.1
656	Gosforth	Copeland	83	10	1.1	12	5.6	3	574	3.8	15.2	2.7	36.9	24.2

No.	Name	District												
587	Belmont	Langbaurgh	106	53	0.6	39	10.7	50	583	7.6	15.7	2.1	16.8	14.4
588	Cleadon and East Boldon	South Tyneside	88	62	1.2	81	10.6	23	661	5.9	17.8	0.7	8.0	5.5
589	Whittingham	Alnwick	87	7	0.4	3	13.8	4	390	6.3	22.2	3.4	68.9	47.1
590	Holker	South Lakeland	129	17	1.4	17	4.3	2	588	5.5	29.0	1.2	28.6	34.4
591	Derwent Valley	Allerdale	131	21	1.7	25	2.4	1	605	6.6	21.8	0.8	33.7	15.9
592	Kendal Fell	South Lakeland	85	10	1.1	10	12.1	7	546	4.9	18.9	1.3	32.7	20.5
593	St. Bees	Copeland	78	10	1.1	13	12.1	6	600	6.8	19.8	1.1	29.2	23.1
594	Binsey	Allerdale	71	10	1.5	20	11.1	1	547	6.2	16.5	2.0	39.3	39.3
595	Cheviot	Berwick-upon-Tweed	83	4	2.7	14	4.5	1	405	4.9	17.8	3.3	80.5	60.0
596	Longhorsley	Castle Morpeth	56	5	1.8	15	11.8	4	559	3.0	17.8	2.6	44.0	10.3
597	Corbridge	Tynedale	89	25	1.7	43	11.8	8	484	3.0	22.1	2.8	43.8	17.5
598	Wark	Tynedale	125	8	1.4	10	3.4	1	543	4.1	21.8	1.3	62.5	14.3
599	Milfield	Berwick-upon-Tweed	72	7	1.6	12	11.9	2	409	5.0	19.7	3.2	77.6	60.6
600	Nunthorpe	Middlesbrough	74	27	0.9	34	11.1	18	657	6.3	5.0	1.4	5.4	11.2
601	Ponteland South	Castle Morpeth	66	18	0.8	19	14.3	6	678	1.9	4.5	0.1	2.1	0.0
602	Millon Without	Copeland	63	6	1.1	16	13.3	6	572	7.0	17.2	1.0	43.9	39.3
603	Kendal Oxenholme	South Lakeland	75	9	1.1	16	11.7	11	666	3.6	19.9	0.7	10.0	31.8
604	Kirkby Lonsdale	South Lakeland	75	11	1.6	23	9.6	5	552	3.9	22.9	2.1	43.7	7.9
605	Kendal Stonecross	South Lakeland	106	15	1.2	17	7.1	5	671	3.2	24.6	0.3	7.4	15.0
606	Chesters	Tynedale	106	9	1.1	9	7.4	2	411	5.8	20.6	3.9	63.0	33.3
607	Cramlington South	Blyth Valley	82	25	0.8	33	11.8	27	632	6.1	19.2	1.2	15.8	14.5
608	Bamburgh	Berwick-upon-Tweed	100	4	1.2	5	7.7	7	415	8.4	33.3	1.4	66.7	26.7
609	Ulverston West	South Lakeland	94	22	0.7	15	10.3	7	638	5.4	21.1	1.3	12.8	15.2
610	Kendal Mintsfeet	South Lakeland	110	14	0.6	8	8.5	8	602	3.6	43.0	1.3	17.9	17.8
611	Broomley and Stocksfield	Tynedale	62	12	1.3	23	12.1	8	640	4.7	22.7	0.9	24.8	10.5
612	Elsdon	Alnwick	85	4	2.2	9	5.3	1	512	3.5	11.9	2.6	68.6	21.4
613	Rothbury	Alnwick	70	13	1.5	26	10.0	5	394	8.9	36.5	2.2	51.8	9.1
614	Fulwell	Sunderland	93	84	1.5	126	10.0	21	563	7.6	36.3	2.2	8.2	8.2
615	North Lodge	Chester-le-Street	74	14	1.2	21	10.4	3	647	4.5	10.6	2.5	6.1	10.5
616	Embleton	Alnwick	69	4	1.1	6	11.5	8	461	7.3	22.7	1.1	64.7	38.9
617	Wetheral	Carlisle	94	25	1.2	30	10.4	6	651	5.9	18.1	0.5	23.4	8.3
618	Holmlands Park	Chester-le-Street	95	13	1.3	33	7.8	6	615	5.6	33.1	1.0	11.7	10.5
619	Kendal Underley	South Lakeland	94	17	1.5	20	11.5	3	422	5.6	39.2	1.7	65.7	22.7
620	Middleton St George	Darlington	100	20	1.8	34	4.3	3	498	7.0	28.9	2.2	32.2	11.5
621	Keswick	Allerdale	77	30	1.5	57	8.4	11	418	9.3	40.6	1.8	44.4	16.2

No.	Ward	District												
552	Staveley in Westmorland	South Lakeland	82	11	2.2	29	9.6	5	581	4.0	27.1	1.7	33.3	15.2
553	Whickham South	Gateshead	89	68	1.3	105	12.4	48	589	6.0	24.4	1.8	18.3	9.7
554	Ulverston South	South Lakeland	109	35	1.3	41	9.7	11	470	6.5	28.6	1.9	50.0	22.6
555	Castle	Tynedale	79	8	1.9	20	11.1	11	378	7.6	40.1	2.6	53.4	18.9
556	Northfield	Stockton-on-Tees	76	36	1.3	54	14.0	20	628	8.2	19.0	1.2	6.1	13.0
557	Egglescliffe	Stockton-on-Tees	74	39	0.8	46	16.2	47	630	6.5	17.5	1.3	14.1	12.8
558	Brotton	Langbaurgh	92	33	2.0	73	8.8	19	358	14.5	33.8	3.9	25.3	24.6
559	Hawcoat	Barrow-in-Furness	96	51	2.0	57	11.1	16	668	3.8	17.7	0.8	2.5	8.2
560	Langwathby	Eden	59	6	1.5	14	15.2	5	590	3.5	19.4	1.8	44.4	19.4
561	Hurworth	Darlington	96	28	1.2	34	11.4	9	629	7.1	21.0	0.7	21.8	11.0
562	Greatham	Hartlepool	81	13	1.4	25	12.6	14	431	11.4	27.7	2.5	35.2	19.7
563	Lyth Valley	South Lakeland	85	10	1.4	16	12.0	6	663	3.2	10.5	0.6	36.6	34.4
564	Burgh	Carlisle	84	17	1.8	30	10.4	7	586	5.3	15.8	1.7	36.9	17.5
565	Penrith West	Eden	96	13	1.4	20	10.1	5	549	5.2	42.4	1.1	29.1	22.2
566	West Dyke	Langbaurgh	80	44	2.0	103	10.1	27	529	11.4	32.4	1.7	4.6	18.0
567	Heskey	Eden	107	20	0.8	14	11.4	8	571	4.5	11.9	1.9	49.4	24.6
568	Kirkoswald	Eden	54	5	1.9	17	13.9	5	528	5.1	14.6	2.8	42.1	4.0
569	Castle	Newcastle upon Tyne	80	73	1.5	137	12.0	58	496	7.7	27.7	2.5	33.8	11.3
570	Whalton	Castle Morpeth	97	7	0.7	5	12.8	6	520	3.3	19.0	2.5	60.6	31.0
571	Amble West	Alnwick	87	14	1.7	29	9.9	10	475	8.4	44.8	1.9	17.2	18.0
572	Brookfield	Middlesbrough	83	37	1.1	59	12.8	42	607	8.3	15.6	3.1	3.1	21.5
573	Dalston	Carlisle	116	24	0.5	18	10.9	6	433	3.5	21.0	0.9	41.1	6.1
574	Burneside	South Lakeland	93	14	1.0	12	11.1	9	658	4.9	32.3	2.4	62.9	11.1
575	Beetham	South Lakeland	68	9	1.0	18	15.2	6	553	5.6	12.4	0.7	18.7	17.2
576	Long Marton	Eden	53	4	2.0	14	13.0	3	553	4.8	18.0	2.5	35.4	23.8
577	Slaley and Hexhamshire	Tynedale	92	7	1.0	14	8.6	3	524	3.7	18.3	2.6	52.9	22.2
578	Acklam	Middlesbrough	93	48	1.6	73	9.2	13	634	8.1	21.1	1.0	6.6	18.0
579	Longframlington	Alnwick	28	2	1.0	11	17.9	5	503	6.7	26.3	1.5	22.3	18.2
580	South Gosforth	Newcastle upon Tyne	104	74	1.0	80	10.2	32	611	6.5	34.2	0.8	42.3	4.1
581	Monkseaton	North Tyneside	69	53	1.5	107	12.5	32	621	6.1	33.8	0.7	15.6	6.9
582	Stanwix Rural	Carlisle	78	27	1.2	40	12.5	16	620	4.8	15.3	1.6	27.1	10.2
583	Ovingham	Tynedale	75	6	1.5	13	11.6	5	562	4.8	25.8	2.0	31.1	9.1
584	St John's Chapel	Wear Valley	96	11	1.4	16	9.1	4	456	11.7	30.9	1.7	30.9	33.3
585	Ponteland West	Castle Morpeth	56	16	1.0	24	15.9	10	677	3.5	5.9	0.3	33.2	3.7
586	Sadberge	Darlington	56	7	1.6	18	13.3	6	593	4.4	20.7	2.0	29.9	17.5

References

Abel-Smith, B. (1967) An international study of health expenditure. World Health Organisation, Geneva, *Public Health Papers, 32*
——— (1979) The cost of health services. *New Society*, 12 July
Adelstein, A.M. and Fox, A.J. (1978) Occupational Mortality: work or a way of life? *Journal of Epidemiology and Community Health, 32*, 73–8
Alma-Ata (1978) *Primary health care. Report of the International Conference on Primary Health Care, Alma-Ata, USSR, 6–12 Sept. 1978*. World Health Organisation, Geneva
Antonovsky, A. (1972) Social class, life expectancy and overall mortality. In E.G. Jaco (ed.), *Patients, physicians and illness*, Free Press, New York
Ashton, J. (1984) *Health in Mersey — a review*. Department of Community Health, University of Liverpool
Beesley, J.R. (1982) *Perinatal mortality in North Tyneside 1976–1981*. North Tyneside Health Authority
Betts, G. (1985) *Health in Glyndon. Report of a survey on health in Glyndon Ward*. Greenwich Resource Centre, Greenwich
Black Report (1980) *Inequalities in health: Report of a Research Working Group*. Department of Health and Social Security, London
Bradshaw, J., Edwards, H., Staden, F. and Weale, J. (1982) Area variations in infant mortality 1975–77. *Journal of Epidemiology and Community Health, 36*, 11–16
Brennan, H.E. and Clare, P.H. (1980) The relationship between mortality and two indicators of morbidity. *Journal of Epidemiology and Community Health, 34*, 134–8
Brennan, M.E. and Lancashire R. (1978) Association of childhood mortality with housing status and employment. *Journal of Epidemiology and Community Health, 32*, 28–33
Brotherston, J. (1976) Inequality: is it inevitable? In C.O. Carter, and J. Peel (eds), *Equalities and inequalities in health*, Academic Press, London
Brown, M. and Madge, N. (1982) *Despite the welfare state*. Heinemann, London
Bryce-Smith, D. (1986) Environmental chemical influences on behaviour and mentation — the John Jeyes lecture. *Chemical Society Reviews, 15*, 93–123
Bulusu, L. (1985) Area mortality comparisons and institutional deaths. *Population trends*, 42, 36–41
Butler, N.R. (1977) Community and family influences on 0 to fives: utilisation of pre-school daycare and preventive health care. Department of Child Health, University of Bristol
Campbell, B. (1984) *Wigan Pier revisited: poverty and politics in the 1980s*. Virago, London
Carr-Hill, R.A. (1985) Health and income: a longitudinal study of four hundred families. *Quarterly Journal of Social Affairs, 4*, 295–307
Carstairs, V. (1982) Health and social deprivation. In A. Smith (ed.), *Recent advances in community medicine*, 2, Churchill Livingstone, Edinburgh, pp. 51–62

Central Statistical Office (1984, 1985, 1986) *Regional Trends, 19, 20,* and *21* respectively, HMSO, London

Centre for Health Studies, Yale University (1977) *A proposal for cooperative multidisciplinary studies of the complex social causation and prevention of ill-health*

Chadwick, E. (1842) *Report on the sanitary condition of the labouring population of Great Britain*

Champion, A. and Green, A. (1985) In search of Britain's booming towns. University of Newcastle-upon-Tyne, Centre for Urban and Regional Development Studies

Charlton, J.R.H., Hartley, R.M., Silver, R. and Holland, W.W. (1983) Geographical variation in mortality from conditions amenable to medical intervention in England and Wales. *The Lancet, 1,* 691–6

────── Baver, R. and Lakhani, A. (1984) Outcome measures for district and regional health care planners. *Community Medicine, 6,* 306–15

────── and Velez, R. (1986) Some international comparisons of mortality amenable to medical intervention. *British Medical Journal, 292,* 295–301

Cole-Hamilton, I. and Lang, T. (1986) *Tightening belts: a report for a working party on food and low income.* London Food Commission

Colley, J.R.T., Douglas, J.W.B. and Reid, D.D. (1973) Respiratory Disease in Young Adults: Influence of Early Childhood Lower Respiratory Tract

Crombie, D.L. (1984) Social class and health status: inequality or difference. *Royal College of General Practitioners, Occasional Papers, 25*

Davie, R., Butler, N. and Goldstein, H. (1972) *From birth to seven: the Second Report of the National Child Development Study (1958 cohort).* Longman, London

Department of Employment (1984, 1985) *Employment Gazette,* HMSO, London

Department of the Environment (1983) Urban Deprivation. *Inner Cities Directorate, Information Note, 2*

Department of Health and Social Security (DHSS) (1976) *Report of the Resource Allocation Working Party.* DHSS, London

────── (1984) *Social Security Statistics.* HMSO, London

Department of Industry (annual) *The investigation of air pollution.* Warren Spring Laboratory

Douglas, J.W.B. (1951) The health and survival of children in different school classes: the results of a national survey. *The Lancet, ii,* 440

────── and Gear, R. (1976) Children of low birthweight in the 1946 national cohort. *Archives of Disease in Childhood, 51,* 820–7

────── and Walker, R.E. (1966) Air pollution and respiratory infection in children. *British Journal of Preventive and Social Medicine, 20,* 1–8

Dubos, R. (1959) *Mirage of health: utopias, progress and biological change.* Harper and Row, New York

Durham County Council (1954) *County Development Plan.* Durham

────── (1969) *County Development Plan First Review.* Durham

Ehrenreich, J. (ed.) (1978) *The cultural crisis of modern medicine.* Monthly Review Press, New York

Engels, F. (1958) *The condition of the working class in England*. Allen and Unwin, London

Eyer, J. and Sterling, P. (1977) Stress-related mortality and social organisation. *Review of Radical Political Economics, 9* (1), 1–44

Farr, W. (1860) On the construction of life tables, illustrated by a new life table of the healthy districts of England. *Journal of the Institute of Actuaries, IX*

Fox, A.J. and Adelstein, A.M. (1978) Occupational mortality: work or a way of life? *Journal of Epidemiology and Community Health, 32,* 73–8

—— and Goldblatt, P.O. (1982) *Longitudinal study: socio-demographic mortality differentials*. HMSO, London, OPCS Series LS No. 1

—— Goldblatt, P.O. and Jones, D.R. (1985) Social class mortality differentials: artefact, selection or life circumstances? *Journal of Epidemiology and Community Health, 39,* 1–8

—— Jones, D.R. and Goldblatt, P.O. (1984) Approaches to studying the effect of socio-economic circumstances on geographic differences in mortality in England and Wales. *British Medical Bulletin, 4,* 309–14

—— and Leon, D.A. (1985) Mortality and deprivation: evidence from the OPCS longitudinal study. *The City University, London, Social Statistics Research Unit, Working Paper, 33*

Goldthorpe, J.H. (1983) Women and class analysis: in defence of the conventional view. *Sociology, 17,* 465–88

—— (1984) Women and class analysis: a reply to the replies. *Sociology, 18,* 491–9

Greater London Council (GLC) (1985) Inner city policy for London: a fresh approach

Halliday, M.L. and Anderson, T. (1979) The sex differential in ischaemic heart disease trends by social class 1931–1971. *Journal of Epidemiology and Community Health, 33,* 74–7

Harrington, J.M. (1978) *Shift work and health: a critical review of the literature*. HMSO, London

Hart, N. (1985) *Sociology of health and medicine*. Causeway Press, London

—— (1986) Inequalities in health: the individual versus the environment. *Journal of the Royal Statistical Society*, Series A, *149* (3), 228–46

Heath, A. and Britten, N. (1984) Women's jobs do make a difference: a reply to Goldthorpe, *Sociology, 18,* 475–490

Health Education Council (HEC) (1987) *The health divide: inequalities in health in the 1980s* prepared by M. Whitehead

Hollingsworth, J.R. (1981) Inequality in levels of health in England and Wales, 1891–1971: *Journal of Health and Social Behaviour, 22* (3), 268–83

Holme, I., Helgeland, A., Hjermann, I., Leren, P. and Lund-Larsen, P.G. (1980) Four year mortality by some socio-economic indicators: the Oslo Study. *Journal of Epidemiology and Community Health, 34,* 48–52

Holterman, S. (1975) Areas of deprivation in Great Britain: an analysis of 1971 Census data. *Social Trends, 6,* 33–47

House of Commons (1980) *Third Report from the Social Services Committee, Session 1979–80. The Government's White Papers on Public Expenditure: The Social Services*. HMSO, London, July 9

Howe, G.M. (1982) London and Glasgow: a spatial analysis of mortality experience in contrasting metropolitan centres. *Scottish Geographical Magazine*, 119–27

Hume, D. and Womersley, J. (1985) Analysis of death rates in the population aged 60 years and over of Greater Glasgow by postcode sector of residence. *Journal of Epidemiology and Community Health, 39*, 357–63

Humphreys, N.A. (1887) Class mortality statistics. *Journal of the Royal Statistical Society, L*

Illich, I. (1975) *Medical nemesis: the appropriation of health.* New York

International Union for the Scientific Study of Population (1984) *Methodologies for the collection and analysis of mortality. Proceedings of conference in Dakar, Senegal, 7–10 July 1981*

Irving, D. and Rice, P. (1984) *Information for health services planning from the 1981 Census.* King's Fund Centre, London

Jarman, B. (1983) Identification of underprivileged areas. *British Medical Journal, 286*, 1705–9

———— (1984) Underprivileged areas: validation and distribution of scores. *British Medical Journal, 289*, 1587–92

———— (1985) Underprivileged areas. In *Medical annual*, John Wright, Bristol

Jones, I.G. and Cameron, D. (1984) Social class analysis — an embarrassment to epidemiology. *Community Medicine, 6*, 37–46

Jones, P. and Cooper, P. (1986) *Inequalities of health in the city of Bristol.* Bristol City Council, Environmental Health Department

Kitagawa, E.M. and Hauser, P.M. (1973) *Differential mortality in the United States.* Harvard University, Cambridge, Mass.

Knox, E.G., Marshall, T., Kane, S., Green, A. and Mallett, R. (1980) Social health care determinants of area variation in perinatal mortality. *Community Medicine, 2*, 282–90

Kosa, J., Antonovsky, A. and Zola, I.K. (eds) (1969) *Poverty and health: a sociological analysis.* Harvard University Press, Cambridge, Mass.

Koskinen, S. (1985) 'Time Trends in Cause-Specific Mortality by Occupational Class in England and Wales'. Department of Sociology, University of Helsinki, paper given to the IUSSP Conference, Florence, Italy

Lalonde, M. (1974) *A new perspective on the health of Canadians.* Minister of Supply and Services, Canada

Lambert, R. (1961) *Sir John Simon.* Cambridge University Press, Cambridge

Lancet editorial (1986) The Occupational Mortality Supplement: why the fuss? Cambridge, *The Lancet, ii*, 610–2

Leavey, R. and Wood, J. (1985) Does the underprivileged area index work? *British Medical Journal, 291*, 709–11

Liaw, K.L., Hayes, M.V. and McAuley, R.G. (1986) Analysis of local mortality variation. *McMaster University, Hamilton, Ontario, Faculty of Social Sciences, Quantitative Studies in Economics and Population, Research Report, 161*

Liverpool City Planning Department (1986) *Health inequalities in Liverpool.* Liverpool

Logan, W.P. (1982) *Cancer mortality by occupation and social class.* HMSO, London, OPCS Studies of Medical and Population Subjects No. 44

McKeown, T. (1971) An historical appraisal of the medical task. In

T. McKeown and McLachlan (eds), *Medical history and medical care*, Oxford University Press, London

—— (1976) *The role of medicine*. Nuffield Provincial Hospitals Trust, London

MacLean, I.H. (1981) Small area analysis and community medicine. Unpublished MSc thesis, University of Newcastle

McMahon, B. and Pugh, T.F. (1970) *Epidemiology: principles and methods*. Little, Brown and Co, New York

Marmot, M.G. (1985) *Social inequalities in mortality — the social environment*. Department of Epidemiology, London School of Hygiene

—— and McDowall, M.E. (1986) Mortality decline and widening social inequalities. The *Lancet, ii*, 274–6

—— Rose, G., Shipley, M. and Hamilton, P.J.S. (1978) Employment grade and coronary heart disease in British civil servants. *Journal of Epidemiology and Community Health, 32*, 244–9

Marsh, G.N. and Channing, D.M. (1986) Deprivation and health in one general practice. *British Medical Journal, 292*, 1173–6

M'Gonigle, G.E.N. and Kirby, J. (1936) *Poverty and public health*. Gollancz, London

Morgan, M. and Chinn, S. (1983) ACORN Group, social class and child health. *Journal of Epidemiology and Community Health, 37*, 196–203

Morris, J.N. (1975) *Uses of epidemiology*. Longman, Edinburgh

Navarro, V. (1976) *Medicine under capitalism*. Prodist, New York

Office of Population Censuses and Surveys (OPCS) (1970) *Classification of occupations*. HMSO, London

—— (1978) *Occupational mortality: Registrar-General's Decennial Supplement, England and Wales, 1970–72*. HMSO, London, Series DS No. 1

—— (1980) *Classification of occupations*. HMSO, London

—— (1981) *Area mortality: Registrar-General's Decennial Supplement, England and Wales, 1969–73*, HMSO, London, Series DS No.4

—— (1981, 1982, 1983) *Vital statistics: local and health areas, England and Wales*. HMSO, London, Series VS, Nos. 8, 9, and 10 respectively

—— (1983) *National report, 1981 Census, Great Britain, Part 1*. HMSO, London

—— (1984) *Census 1981. Key statistics for urban areas: the North cities and towns*. HMSO, London

—— (1986) *Occupational mortality: Decennial Supplement 1979–80, 1982–83, Great Britain*. HMSO, London

Orr, J.B. (1936) *Food, health and income*

Palmer, S., West, P., Patrick, D. and Glynn, M. (1979) Mortality indices in resource allocation. *Community Medicine, 1*, 275–81

Pamuk, E.R. (1985) Social class inequality in mortality from 1921 to 1972 in England and Wales. *Population Studies, 39*, 17–31

Paterson, K. (1981) Theoretical perspectives in epidemiology — a critical appraisal. *Radical Community Medicine, 8*, 21–9

Piachaud, D. (1986) Disability, retirement and unemployment of older men. *Journal of Social Policy, 15* (2), 145–62

Powles, J. (1973) On the limitations of modern medicine. *Science, Medicine and Man, 1*, 1–30

203

——— Registrar General (1842) *Fifth Annual Report, 1841*. HMSO, London

——— (1875) *Supplement to the Thirty-fifth Annual Report*. HMSO, London

——— (1950, 1951, 1952) *Statistical Review of England and Wales, Part 1, Medical*. HMSO, London

Rogers, G.B. (1979) Income and inequality as determinants of mortality: an international cross section analysis. *Population Studies, 33,* 343–51

Rose, G. and Marmot, M.G. (1981) Social class and coronary heart disease. *British Heart Journal, 45,* 13–19

Rosen, G. (1958) *A history of public health*. MD Publications, New York

Salonen, J.T. (1982) Socio-economic status and risk of cancer, cerebral stroke and death due to coronary heart disease and any disease: a longitudinal study in eastern Finland. *Journal of Epidemiology and Community Health, 36,* 294–7

Saull, H. (1983) *Occupational mortality in 1971–75*. Central Statistical Office of Finland, Studies, No. 54, Helsinki

Scott-Samuel, a. (1983) Identification of underprivileged areas. *British Medical Journal, 287,* 130

——— (1984) Need for primary health care: an objective indicator. *British Medical Journal, 288,* 457–8

——— (1986) Social inequalities in health: back on the agenda. *The Lancet, i,* 1084–5

Seabrook, J. (1985) *Landscapes of poverty*. Blackwell, Oxford

Sheffield Health Authority (1986) *Health care and disease: a profile of Sheffield*. Sheffield

Simanis, J.G. (1973) Medical care expenditure in seven countries. *Social Security Bulletin,* March

Skrimshire, A. (1978) *Area disadvantage, social class and the health service*. University of Oxford, Department of Social and Administrative Studies

Smail, R. (1985) *Two nations: poverty wages in the North*. Newcastle Low Pay Unit

Stacey, M. (1977) Concepts of health and illness: a working paper on the concepts and their relevance for research. In *Health and health policy — priorities for research*, the report of an advisory panel to the Research Initiatives Board, London, Social Science Research Council, May

Stanworth, M. (1984) Women and class analysis: a reply to John Goldthorpe. *Sociology, 18,* 159–70

Stark, E. (1982) Doctors in spite of themselves: the limits of radical health criticism. *International Journal of Health Services, 12* (3), 419–55

Stevenson, T.H.C. (1923) The social distribution of mortality from different causes in England and Wales 1910–1912. *Biometrika, XV*

——— (1928) The vital statistics of wealth and poverty. *Journal of the Royal Statistical Society, XCI,* 207–30

Susser, M. (1962) Civilisation and peptic ulcer. *The Lancet, 1,* 115–19

Syme, S.L. and Berkman, L.F. (1976) Social class, susceptibility and sickness. *American Journal of Epidemiology, 104,* 1–8

Szreter, S.R.S. (1984) The genesis of the Registrar-General's social classification of occupations. *British Journal of Sociology, 35,* 522–46

Thunhurst, C.P. (1985a) *Poverty and health in the city of Sheffield*. Environmental Health Department, City of Sheffield, pp. 93–16

—— (1985b) The analysis of small area statistics and planning for health. *The Statistician, 34*, 93–106

Titmuss, R.M. (1938) *Poverty and population.* Macmillan, London

Townsend, P. (1979) *Poverty in the United Kingdom.* Penguin, Harmondsworth, Middlesex

—— (1987) Deprivation. *Journal of Social Policy*, April

—— Corrigan, P. and Kowarzik, U. (1987) *Poverty and labour in London: interim report of a Centenary Survey.* Low Pay Unit, London

—— and Davidson, N. (eds) (1982) *Inequalities in health (the Black Report).* Penguin, Harmondsworth, Middlesex

—— Simpson, D. and Tibbs, N. (1984) *Inequalities of health in the City of Bristol.* Department of Social Administration, University of Bristol

Tyne and Wear County Council (1985) *Unemployment in Tyne and Wear*

Uemura, K. and Pisa, Z. (1985) Recent trends in cardiovascular disease mortality in 27 industrialised countries. *World Health Statistical Quarterly, 38*, 142

UK Government (1980) *The Government's White Papers on Public Expenditure: the Social Services. Reply by the Government to the Third Report from the Social Services Committee.* HMSO, London, Session 1979–80, Cmnd 8086

United Nations (1984) *Socio-economic differential mortality in industrialised societies, Vol. 3, proceedings of meeting in Rome 24–27 May, 1983.* WHO-CICRED

Valkonen, T. (1982) Socio-economic mortality differentials in Finland. *University of Helsinki, Department of Sociology, Working Paper, 28*

Virchow, R. (ed. Rather, L.J.) (1958) *Disease, life and man: selected essays of Rudolf Virchow.* Stanford University Press

Wadsworth, M.E.J. and Morris, S. (1978) Assessing chances of hospital admission in pre-school children: a critical evaluation. *Archives of Disease in Childhood, 53*, 159–63

Webber, R. (1977) *The classification of residential neighbourhoods: an introduction to the classification of wards and parishes.* Centre for Environmental Studies, London, PRAG Technical Report TP 23

West of Scotland Politics of Health Group (1984) *Glasgow, health of a city*

Wilkinson, R.G. (1976) *'Socio-economic differentials in mortality'.* M. Med Sci thesis

—— (1986a) Socio-economic differences in mortality: interpreting the data on their size and trends. In R.G. Wilkinson (ed.), *Class and health: research and longitudinal data*, Tavistock, London

—— (1986b) Income and mortality. In R.G. Wilkinson (ed.) *Class and health: research and longitudinal data*, Tavistock, London

Winter, J.M. (1977) The impact of the First World War on civilian health in Britain. *Economic History Review, 30*, 487–507

—— (1981) Aspects of the impact of the First World War on infant mortality in Britain. *Journal of European Economic History, 11*, 713–38

World Health Organisation Regional Office for Europe (1984) *Health promotion — a discussion document on the concept and principles.* WHO, Copenhagen

Index

Page references in *italics* refer to tables or figures. Page references incorporating 'n' refer to notes.

age
  and death rate 25, *26–7*, 58–60, *85*, 86, *130–2*
  and deprivation 35
Allerdale
  deprivation 72
  mortality 49
Alnwick
  deprivation 70
  ill-health in 47
  mortality 49
anorexia nervosa 14
asbestos 14
Ashington, mortality 55

Barrow-in-Furness
  deprivation 70
    and low birthweight 110
  ill-health in 47
Berwick-upon-Tweed
  deprivation 70
  ill-health in 47
  mortality 49, 52, 55
birth registration records 163
birthweight, low 30, 31, 32, *62–5*
  and class *101*, 102
  associated with deprivation 107, *108*, 110–11, *173*
  'excess' 155
  reflection of present conditions 33
Black Report, The 16–17, 161
  factors determining class 140
  interpretation of class 10, 95–6
  models of health 6
  widening inequalities in health 151
Black Research Working Group 128, 132–3, 140, 141

Blue Hall estate 64, 159n4

cadmium 15
carcinogens, mapped 14
Carlisle, ill-health in 47
car ownership *169*
  and deprivation 36, 37, 73, 153, 156
  and health 77, 107, *108*, 117, *118*, 120
Castle Morpeth
  deprivation 70
  ill-health in 47
  mortality 49
Census Small Area Statistics (1981) 36, 71, 163
cholera 3
civil servants, mortality 5
class
  interpretation of 10–11, 95–6
  occupational 11, 95–6
    and deprivation 38, 66, 116, *118*, 119–21, *177*, *178*
    and health 4–6, 34
    and low birthweight *101*, 102
    and mortality 96–*100*, 102, 128–39, 155–6, 157–8
    and mortality ratios 23, *25*, 128–*30*
  female 96–7
  measuring 144
  widening differences between 128
Cleveland
  deprivation 66, 70
  low birthweight in 62, 64, *65*
  mortality *49–50*, *51*, *105–6*, 121–7, 157

avoidable *176*
unemployment 70–1, 159n5
urban areas 167
see also Hartlepool
Copeland
deprivation 72
ill-health in 47
mortality 49
permanent sickness 62
Cumbria
permanent sickness 62
urban areas 167
see also West Cumbria

Darlington
ill-health in 47
mortality 47, 49
death registration records 163
deaths *see* mortality
decennial supplements on
mortality 4, 128, 140, 161
*Occupational mortality:
decennial supplement*
(1986) 128, 143–4
Department of Health, health
care policies 12–13
deprivation
linked to health 74–91,
107–27, 116–21, 155,
172, 176, 177
linked to mortality 121–7
measuring 34–8, 153 *see also*
'overall deprivation index'
prevalence 66–73
urban and rural 72–3, *78, 79*
deprivation index *see* 'overall
deprivation index'
Derwentside
deprivation 66, 72
permanent sickness 60
development, delayed 31 *see
also* birthweight, low
diet
and social factors 13–14
zinc deficiency 14–15
disability *see* sickness,
permanent
district health authorities,
population sizes 38
Dubos, R. 9

Durham
deprivation 72–3
linked to health 115
female mortality *53*, 54
permanent sickness 60, 62
unemployment 71
urban areas 167
see also Darlington

Easington 45
deprivation 66, 70, 72
and low birthweight 113
life in pit villages 89–91
poor health 153, 154
amongst rural communities
115
low birthweight 62
mortality 47, 49, 52
permanent sickness 60
Eden
deprivation 70
mortality 49
ethnicity, and deprivation 35

family solidarity, and health 15
Farr, William 139

Gateshead
deprivation 66
mortality 50, *51*, 52, 106,
124, 154
permanent sickness 60
Guildford
mortality *26*, 27
unemployment 29

Hartlepool
deprivation 66, 70
ill-health in 45
low birthweight 64, 110
mortality 47, 50, 52, 53,
106, 124
health
and social class 4–6
Government expenditure on
12–13
in different areas 43–7,
179–98
history 3–4
reasons for unequal 98–9

shown by low birthweight
62–5, 152, 164
shown by mortality 47–60,
152, 163
shown by sickness 60–2,
152, 163
linked to deprivation 74–91,
107–27, 155, *172*, *176*,
177
measuring 30–3, 152 *see also*
'overall health index'
research into 3–4, 16–17
social and medical models
6–11
health care policies 12–13, 14,
15–17
health index *see* 'overall health
index'
home ownership *171*
and deprivation 36, 37, 73,
153
and health 77, *118*, 119
House of Commons Social
Services Committee, quoted
on health expenditure 12
Howdon 58, 59, 60
Hutton 153, 154

income
and class 11
reflected by occupation 140–1
variation within occupations 5

Lancet, The
editorial on class inequalities
145
editorial on social class
143–4
Langbaurgh
deprivation 71
ill-health in 47, 153
linked to deprivation 111
mortality 50, 52, 124, 154
'excess' 106
unemployment 71
lead 14, 15
life tables 139
living standards, North and
South 27–9
local authority areas

health and deprivation 34–5,
79, *80–1*, 159n2
sizes 38
London
deprivation and the North
34–5, 73
mortality ratios 25

Medizinische Reform (Virchow) 9
Merseyside, unemployment 71
M'Gonigle, G.C.M. and Kirby,
J. 18, 158
Middlesbrough
deprivation 66, 70, 124
ill-health in 45, 47
linked with deprivation
111, 156
low birthweight in 62
mortality *26*, 27, 47, 50, 52,
124
'excess' 106
permanent sickness 60
unemployment 27, 71
mobility, social 4–5, 6
Monkseaton 59, 91
mortality 20, 22–3, *24*, 47–60
and deprivation 84–6, 121–7,
174
avoidable *175*, *176*
causes 55, *56*, 86–8, 99,
100, 102
and class 133–9
changing trends 25
civil servant 5
class differences in 5–6,
96–*100*, 102, 128–39, 149
Registrar General's
approach 139–45, 149
the North compared with
Britain 145–9
compared to other countries
20, *21*, 22–3
data from private households
164
distribution by age 25–7
estimating 166
'excess' 84, *146*, 154
and occupational class
102–6
in Britain *146*, 147

England and Wales 26–7, 57, 58–9
part of a health index 31–2, 33
see also standard mortality ratios

Newcastle-upon-Tyne
children's health in the 1930s 18–19
deprivation 66
linked to health 114–15
mortality 50, 51, 52, 106, 124, 154
permanent sickness 60
unemployment 71
noise 14
North of England
economy 19–20, 159n1
population geography 19
populations within authorities 38
North-South divide 25–9
North Tyneside
deprivation, and low birthweight 110
low birthweight in 64
mortality 58–60, 106, 124, 155
Northumberland
mortality 55, 57
urban areas 167

occupation see class, occupational
OPCS 161
data derived from 163
mortality data see decennial supplements on mortality
'overall deprivation index' 165
linked to health 107–12, 155
measures for 36–7, 156–7
'overall health index' 165
and class 116, 118, 119–21
linked to deprivation 107–12, 116–19, 155
measures for 30–3, 152
wards ranked by 43, 179–98
overcrowding 170

and deprivation 36, 37, 73, 153
and health 77, 118, 119

parenthood, single, and deprivation 35
parliamentary constituencies, health and deprivation 79, 82–3, 84
pit villages, Easington 89–91
pollution, as an index of deprivation 126–7, 157
population
local authority 38
North of England 19
Poverty and public health (M'Gonigle and Kirby) 18–19
prosperity, in the North 19–20, 159n1

redundancies 29
Registrar General 161
approach to mortality/class relationship 139–45, 149
classification of class 10–11, 95–6, 161
decennial supplements on mortality 4, 128, 140, 143–4, 161
regression analysis
for health inequality 116–21
for mortality differences 121–7
Report of the Resource Allocation Working Party (DHSS) 3
Report of the Working Group on Inequalities in Health see Black Report
Riverside 58, 59, 60
rural communities, county planning designations 115

St Mary's 59, 91
sexes, and mortality 52–3, 55, 57, 84
Shotton, 89, 90
sickness, permanent 30, 31, 32, 33, 60–2

associated with deprivation
107, *108*, *172*
distribution in Britain *22*, 23
'excess' 154–5
smoking 138
Snow, John 3
Southern England, mortality
ratios *24*
South Lakeland
deprivation 70
ill-health in 47
mortality 49
permanent sickness 62
South Tyneside
deprivation 70, 72, 113
ill-health in 47
linked to deprivation 113
low birthweight 65, 113
mortality 50
unemployment 71
standardised mortality ratios
(SMRs) *25*, 30–1, 161–2
by region of Britain *148*
cause of death *56*, 57, 86–8
and class 133–9
for occupational class 103,
104
meaning 161–2
see also mortality
Stockton
deprivation 66, 70
low birthweight in 62, 64
mortality 124
during 1928–32 18
stress 15
Sunderland
deprivation 70
ill-health in 47
linked to deprivation 111,
156
low birthweight in 64, 65
mortality 50, 155
'excess' 106
permanent sickness 60
unemployment 71

Teesdale
low birthweight in 62, 64
mortality 49
Teesside

air pollution 126, 127
unemployment 71
Thornley 89, 90
Tyne and Wear
deprivation 66, 70
low birthweight in 64–*5*
mortality *49*–50, 121–7, 157
avoidable *176*
unemployment 71, 159n5
Tynedale
ill-health in 47
mortality 49

unemployment 19–20, *168*
and health 77, 107, *108*, 117,
118, 119
and living standards 5
measure of deprivation 36,
70–2, 73, 153
urban areas
definition 167
deprivation in *78*, 79

vinyl chloride 14
Virchow, Rudolf 9

wards
best and worst for health 43,
179–98
changed boundaries 40
clustering 39
and low birthweight 65
and mortality 50–7, 124–6
local authority 38–40
overall health in 45–7
rural *78*, 79
urban *78*, 79
Wear Valley
deprivation 66, 72
ill-health in 45
mortality 53
permanent sickness 60
West Cumbria
areas of high mortality *54*–5
deprivation 72, 73
Wheatley Hill *44*, 89, 90,
153–4
Whitley Bay, affluent areas of
91
Wingate 89, 90

women
classified by husbands'
occupation 142
mortality 52–3, 55, 57, 84
gradients of 142
in areas of Britain 146,
147
relationship to class 96–7,
130, 131–2, 136–7,
145–8
wage-earning and
occupational class 141

World Health Organization
(WHO)
definition of health 9
reduction in health inequality
158

Yale University, Centre for
Health Studies 13–14,
15–16

zinc deficiency 14–15
Z-scores technique 33, 165